Surgical Talk
Surgery for Finals

Surgical Talk
Surgery for Finals

Andrew Goldberg

FRCS(Eng), FRCSI
Specialist Registrar in Trauma & Orthopaedics
Stanmore Royal National Orthopaedic Hospital
Stanmore, Middlesex, UK

Gerard Stansby

Professor of Vascular Surgery
Newcastle University and Freeman Hospital
Newcastle, UK

Imperial College Press

Published by

Imperial College Press
57 Shelton Street
Covent Garden
London WC2H 9HE

Distributed by

World Scientific Publishing Co. Pte. Ltd.
5 Toh Tuck Link, Singapore 596224
USA office: Suite 202, 1060 Main Street, River Edge, NJ 07661
UK office: 57 Shelton Street, Covent Garden, London WC2H 9HE

British Library Cataloguing-in-Publication Data
A catalogue record for this book is available from the British Library.

First published 1999
Reprinted 2002, 2004

SURGICAL TALK: SURGERY FOR FINALS

ISBN   1-86094-077-3
ISBN   1-86094-206-7 (pbk)

Printed in Great Britain by Athenaeum Press Ltd.

CONTENTS

FOREWORD

The authors are to be congratulated on a clearly written and presented text. Using this book the student can build up a firm foundation of both knowledge and skills, which will not only enable the hurdle of finals to be negotiated with confidence, but will also be of everyday value in clinical practice.

Visually attractive, readable and scientifically sound, the book makes relatively light work of the large volume of information contained within.

It seems likely to me that this book will appeal not only to students with final examinations in mind, but also to house surgeons and senior house officers with patients to diagnose and treat and, perhaps, with the MRCS on the horizon.

Professor Averil Mansfield, CBE, ChM, FRCS

PREFACE

When you are a medical student, finals seem a daunting prospect. However, the truth is that most candidates pass the exam easily and most junior doctors look back at finals as being relatively straightforward. The reason for this is that this exam is simply the last hurdle in a long and draining race and by the time you have reached this point the odds are with you to finish the course. The examiners are not there to fail candidates per se; in fact, the opposite is true and they are really trying to help you pass. However, they must ensure that a safe junior doctor is unleashed on the public. Because of this fact you must know the basics of all the common emergency situations. Luck plays only a small part in finals for most students and, as someone once said, "The harder you work, the luckier you get."

The philosophy of this book is to focus on the level of knowledge and the approach that would be expected of the better students arriving at finals. We have tried to include as much as possible without making the book too cumbersome. No book of this scope can include every possible topic, but we hope that we have included all that could legitimately be expected of you for the final exam. The book also contains comprehensive sections on trauma, orthopaedics and urology, which so often get left out of other texts, and a section on fluid balance that may continue to be of use when you are a junior house officer.

The text has been deliberately written in a tutorial-like story format as opposed to a set of lists, since this makes it easier to understand and remember. Everyone loves a list but we must assure you that you are much more likely to remember a list if you have written it yourself. Therefore, space has been left adjacent to the text for you to pick out important details from the text and jot down your own lists. If you do this as you go along you will effectively produce your own textbook which will become an invaluable tool, with all you need for success at your fingertips.

Good luck with your revision and the exam, and we hope this book will help.

Andrew Goldberg
Gerard Stansby

ACKNOWLEDGMENTS

Marie Stansby, for her help with the illustrations.

Mr. *Jonathan Glass*, Consultant Urologist, Guys & St. Thomas's Hospital NHS Trust, London, UK, for his major contribution to the section on urology.

The *American College of Surgeons* Committee on Trauma, for their kind permission to use the ATLS® principles.

All the *medical students*, for their suggestions before, whilst and after the book was written.

1

SURGICAL TALK

There is no doubt that the best performers in finals are those candidates who think logically, express themselves clearly and avoid putting their foot in their mouth by saying something stupid. Their depth of knowledge is not necessarily greater than that of their fellow candidates, but they do well in every part of the exam — writtens, clinicals and the viva.

The message is clear: you must start early, practising a systematic approach to the subject. In this chapter several examples of such approaches are given. You may not like all of them, so choose a method that you can use and spend a great deal of time perfecting it. Also note that a short pause before answering does not detract from the answer and may avoid a dreadful mistake.

Remember also that in finals the examiners are looking for a minimum standard across the breadth of medicine and surgery. Effectively they wish to assess whether you will be safe as a house officer subsequently. They will not be impressed by superb knowledge in one area if there is ignorance about basic facts in another. You will not be expected to know the technical details of any particular operation but should have an understanding of the broad principles and common complications that would be explained to the patient. An example question might be "What would you say to the patient when consenting him for this operation?"; if you did not know that there were two incisions or that there was a high chance of needing a colostomy, then how could you be expected to inform the patient correctly?

It follows that it is in your best interest to make sure that you know the essential basics about all relevant topics before attempting to learn some topics in greater detail. It is also a basic fact of human psychology that, when revising, students tend to revise more often the areas they feel comfortable about. In fact it is the areas you feel uncomfortable about that you need to spend time on. To avoid leaving gaps in your revision take the chapter headings of your surgical textbook and make sure that you feel you could give a short summary of the basic points in each chapter. If you cannot say much about a particular subject (and would dread being asked about it in finals), then that is your most urgent revision priority — do not leave it to chance.

SURGICAL SIEVES

Sometimes you are asked an obscure question which throws you. Your mind goes blank, you blurt out the first thing that comes into your head, and you end up in a deep hole, especially as you probably do know the answer, or at least some of it anyway. A sieve allows you to gather your thoughts, working from first principles, and come up with at least some sensible statements. When you answer a question you should really talk about the most common things first and the rarities at the end, and one disadvantage of using a sieve is that you may not be able to rapidly reorganize your thoughts in this way, but still it is useful when all else fails and is invaluable in essay writing.

The Aetiological Sieve

- Congenital
- Acquired
- Traumatic
- Inflammatory (physical, chemical, infected)
- Neoplastic (benign or malignant, primary or secondary)
- Circulatory
- Autoimmune
- Nutritional
- Metabolic
- Endocrine

- Drugs
- Degenerative
- Iatrogenic
- Psychosomatic

TIN CAN MED DIP is one way of remembering it, but you probably have your own version.

The Anatomical Sieve

This can apply to anatomical sites, structures or tissue types. If asked "What are the causes of mechanical bowel obstruction?", you could say "Adhesions!". This is a correct answer but an incorrect way of saying it. Start by saying that the bowel is a structure consisting of several regions and hence obstruction can occur anywhere along its length. Then divide it anatomically into stomach outflow obstruction, small bowel obstruction and large bowel obstruction. The examiner will then usually pick one route and lead you along it. If writing an essay you obviously need to discuss all three.

Then add that the bowel is a hollow tube, and like any hollow tube (cf. ureters) it can become blocked at three sites: from outside the tube pressing in (extramural), within the wall of the tube (intramural) and within the lumen of the tube (luminal). Where appropriate, answers should be structured in this way.

Causes of Mechanical Bowel Obstruction:

Extramural	Intramural	Luminal
Adhesions	Tumours	Impacted faeces
Strangulated hernia	Infarction	Foreign body
Volvulus	Strictures	Large polyps
Extrinsic compression	Inflammation	Intussusception

Tissue Types

Try to list the causes of a lump in the groin. It is difficult to be exhaustive. A good method is to say that this lump can arise from any of the tissue types in this region. For example:

Tissue type	Example
Skin	Sebaceous cyst or lipoma
Connective tissue	Fibroma
Lymphatics	Enlarged lymph node
Blood vessels	Saphena varix, femoral artery aneurysm
Inguinal canal	Inguinal hernia, hydrocoele of the cord
Femoral canal	Femoral hernia
Testes	Undescended testes

Do not forget that there are other structures such as muscle, bone, joints and nerves in the region, but in this case these would rarely be the cause. If possible, when listing differential diagnoses try to do so in the order of their likelihood (i.e. do not mention vanishingly rare things before common things).

General and Specific

"Tell me about postoperative complications." When asked such a question it is difficult to know where to start. As before, you must avoid saying the first thing that comes into your head, as this may not be the most relevant.

Here we can use two types of classification: one applies to the type of complication, and the other gives a time scale. Postoperative complications can be *generalized*, i.e. applying to any operation (such as the effects of anaesthesia), or *specific*, i.e. applying to this operation (such as damage to the recurrent laryngeal nerve in thyroidectomy).

Once classified into general and specific the complications can be broken down further into time scales. These complications can be *immediate*, *early* or *late* (see chapter on pre- and postoperative complications for further details).

Once you use these principles, it becomes easy to answer most questions logically. For example: "What are the causes of haematuria?" The causes can be *generalized* (e.g. a bleeding disorder, or use of anticoagulants) or *specific* causes relating to any of the anatomical structures in the region. The following structures (starting from the top) are part of the urinary tract:

Structure	*Cause*
Kidney	Stones, trauma, carcinoma (use the aetiological sieve)
Ureter	Tumours, stones, infection
Bladder	Infection, tumour, stones
Prostate	Benign hypertrophy, tumour, infection
Urethra	Stone, infection, trauma, etc.

NB. Confirm true haematuria, since the appearance of red urine without any blood actually present could be due to beetroot ingestion, or drugs such as rifampicin. Also exclude bleeding from the vagina or anus.

Investigations

Always break down investigations in the following manner:

(1) *Simple urine and faecal tests* (e.g. urine dipstix, microscopy & culture, pregnancy tests, faecal occult blood).
(2) *Haematological tests* (routine, e.g. FBC; or special, e.g. tumour markers).
(3) *Radiological tests* (e.g. CXR, ultrasound or CT).
(4) *Special investigations* (e.g. gastroscopy, V/Q scans).

It is easy to shout out "Full blood count", "Chest X-ray" or "Calcium" as an answer to the question "How would you investigate such a patient?". However, if you think of and say the above list every time you answer such a question, going through the categories one by one, you will never leave out something by mistake. You may be asked to justify your choice of investigation. Often we send off investigations as a baseline since the patients are being admitted to hospital. This is justified in the elderly but is usually a waste of resources in young, fit patients. A full blood count is justified in young females, to check for anaemia. U & E's should be sent for patients on diuretics.

Management

"Discuss the treatment of benign prostatic hypertrophy" is a different question from "Discuss the management of benign prostatic hypertophy". In the former the examiners want you to purely concentrate on treatment and not on diagnosis. In your answer you should define BPH and perhaps say one or two sentences on the condition and its investigation, but do not spend too long on this as you will get no extra marks. Management involves discussing all of the steps that deal with a clinical problem, including the history, examination, investigations, formation of a diagnosis and treatment.

When discussing treatment you can again break down your answer into subheadings. For example:
Treatment can be conservative, medical or surgical. For example, in this case:

Conservative. This usually means ruling out cancer. A prostate specific antigen (PSA) < 4 and a normal examination would help the doctor reassure the patient and a policy of watchful waiting may be adopted until the symptoms get worse.

Medical. For example, drugs such as $\alpha 1$ adreno-receptor blockers or 5-α-reductase inhibitors.

Surgical. For example, trans-urethral resection of the prostate (TURP).

Answering an Essay

Essay questions nowadays tend to be quite generalized; for example, "Minimal access surgery — discuss." However, there will always be the odd question based on a detailed knowledge of one condition.

The following is a guide for the headings you can use in writing such an essay; some surgeons refer to this as the pathological sieve.

- Definition
- Aetiology (incidence, age, sex, geography)/risk factors
- Histology (macro and micro)
- Clinical features (signs and symptoms)
- Diagnosis (and differential)
- Clinical staging (if appropriate)
- Investigations/treatment/management
- Complications
- Prognosis

Remember that "management depends on diagnosis" and that "diagnosis depends on history, examination and special investigations". Therefore "management" refers to all of the steps of clinical assessment and investigation as well as treatment.

Never forget the steps of management which occur early on as the patient is being admitted to hospital. For example, if asked how you would manage a case of acute cholecystitis, you need to say that you would give the patient adequate analgesia, arrange admission to a surgical bed, put up a drip, keep nil by mouth, etc., before talking about liver function tests or ultrasound scans (which would not normally be available immediately). It is often a good idea to try and imagine that you are actually the doctor in A & E who is trying to sort the patient out. What would you actually do? What observations would you ask the nurses to take? When would you review the patient? Would you inform someone more senior? Would you put in a urinary catheter, etc.? By mentioning such points you not only increase the content of your answer, you also demonstrate that you have become aware of the practical aspects of being a junior doctor as well as of the textbook theory.

As part of your management always add the word "POSSET" at the end of an essay — *P*hysio, *O*ccupational therapy, *S*pecialists (e.g. stoma care, breast care, speech therapists), *S*ocial workers, *E*ducation and *T*erminal care. The last two are of utmost importance. Education involves explaining when the stitches will come out, what you can and cannot do, (such as when you can drive, have sex), etc. Terminal care means involving the Macmillan Nurses, arranging the syringe pump to deliver analgesia, speaking to the GP, etc. This last paragraph can be the difference between a good essay and an excellent one.

History of a Lump

There are only five questions you need to remember when taking the history of a lump:

- When and how did you first notice the lump?
- How has the lump changed since you first noticed it?
- What symptoms does it cause you?
- Have you got any more or have you had this before?
- What do you think it is?

You must learn this list. These are the vital questions and they apply to any lump, whether it be in the neck, in the breast or in the groin.

For example, was it *noticed* incidentally, whilst looking in the mirror, or did your partner point it out to you? Remember that this is when the lump was first noticed and not when it first appeared!

How has it changed? Has it got bigger, smaller, stayed the same size, or has it come and gone? Has it changed its appearance and consistency, does it get bigger during her period?, etc.

What symptoms? Is it painful? (patients often wrongly equate this to cancer). For breast lumps, is there a nipple discharge? A lump in the neck could affect voice, respiration or eating. If you think this is a thyroid lump, ask relevant questions about hypo- or hyperthyroidism.

Have you got any more/had it before? If the patient has many lumps, are they the same? If he has had this before, what happened to it the last time, and what did the doctor say it was? Does it come periodically (for example with every menstrual cmycle)?

What do you think it is? This is an important question, since the answer may be "Cancer doctor". You are then aware of the patient's anxieties. You may be able to reassure him even if you do not know the exact diagnosis. For example, you may reassure a 20-year-old girl with a painful breast lump that breast cancer is rare at this age and usually is not painful, etc. This in fact allows you to say something despite not knowing the exact diagnosis yet.

History of a Pain

Again there are only a few questions you need to remember:

- Where is the pain?
- What is the nature of the pain?
- How did the pain start and what has happened to it since?
- What relieves and what exacerbates the pain?
- Are there any associated symptoms?
- Have you ever had this before? / previous history.
- What do you think it is?

As seen with the history of a lump, this set of questions can apply to any pain, whether cardiac in origin or due to appendicitis.

Site. Remember that visceral pain is referred along the somatic nerves; for example, diaphragmatic irritation is felt at the shoulder, and early appendicitis is felt around the umbilicus.

Nature. This includes character, severity and radiation. Colicky pains feel like the contents of a tube are being squashed or pushed forwards. They originate from a hollow viscus, and usually come and go in a regular pattern. Severity is difficult to standardize, since everyone has a different threshold of pain, but saying something like "The pain is worse than labour pains" or "This is the worst pain I've ever had" usually suffices for the meaning.

What has happened to the pain? This includes onset, progression and end. Was the onset sudden or gradual? Has the pain got better or worse since it started? Does it come and go? How is it now compared to when it started? I often get the patient to draw a graph of the pain against time.

Asking the patient for *aggravating or relieving factors* often leads to a blank and you may have to ask more direct questions in this context. For example, does the pain want to make you writhe about or lie very still? Classically, colicky pains make you move about trying to get comfortable, whereas if there is inflammation involving the peritoneum then moving about makes the pain worse. This distinction is helpful in differentiating biliary colic, where the patient may be moving about during an episode, from cholecystitis, where the patient will tend to lie still.

Associated symptoms. Again this will depend on the cause and site of the pain. For example, nausea and vomiting and signs of sympathetic stimulation all go with cardiac pain. Anorexia, weight loss, change in the bowel habit and maybe rectal bleeding would be suggestive of a bowel cancer, etc.

Past history. If the patient has had this pain before he can usually tell you if this feels the same as the last episode — for example an alcoholic with repeated episodes of acute pancreatitis, or the angina sufferer, with an MI. Ask about the past medical history and what drugs the patient is taking.

Answering a Question

By the time finals come along, almost everyone knows how to answer a viva question with the boring words "I would take a thorough history, examine the patient and investigate according to my findings…"

The examiner hears this statement time after time after time, and when the candidate cannot back it up with something more substantial, the examiner rightly becomes annoyed.

A better approach which will make you stand out from the rest of the candidates is to apply your answer directly to the question. So if for example you are asked how you would manage someone with a breast lump, you could say, "In my history I would find out about the history of the lump and ask in particular for risk factors for breast cancer or for factors suggestive of benign breast disease.... On examination I would inspect the breasts, followed by palpation, examining the normal side first, etc.... My investigations would then be tailored to my findings from the history and examination, but should involve an imaging technique plus or minus a fine needle aspiration. The patient would then require counselling about the disease, and treatment could be divided into medical and surgical options (which can be subdivided into curative and palliative)."

This is not meant to give you the full answer — it only highlights the approach you would use (the correct answer is in the chapter on breast surgery). It is clear that this answer shows that you are thinking properly and not merely giving stereotypical responses.

If the examiner wants to test you further he may then go on, "Good, so tell me what questions you would like to know in taking the history of this lump", or "What are the risk factors for breast cancer?" This way you are forcing the examiner into asking you questions that you want to hear, and hence you are always one step ahead.

Likewise, if the examiner asks you for the complications of thyroidectomy, do not spend too much time on the general complications; rather, use perhaps a simple sentence like "Any operation has both general and specific complications and each can be divided into immediate, early and late. The specific complications of thyroidectomy are ...". If he wishes to know the general complications he can then ask you — this way it shows that you understand the question being asked.

It may be possible to give an adequate performance even when you are unsure of the exact diagnosis. A clear history or good clinical examination technique will go a long way towards persuading the examiners that you should pass. Often, if you have accurately reported the history and physical signs, the examiners will give you a hint towards the correct diagnosis if you do not get it immediately.

2

FLUID BALANCE AND PARENTERAL NUTRITION

I can almost guarantee that during your first night on call as a surgical house officer you will be asked to write up IV fluids.

It is important to understand fluid balance, which is best learnt from first principles; unfortunately, this is a subject that is poorly covered in most texts.

BASIC FACTS

The human body is composed of approximately two-thirds water. The contribution of water to body weight depends on how much fat you carry. This is because fat contains very little water. As you age you gain fat and also women tend to have a greater proportion of fat, and therefore women and the elderly will have a smaller proportion of total body water.

If we say body water is 60% of our weight, then a 70 kg man will have 42 l water. Of this 42 l, two-thirds (28 l) will be intracellular (ICF), and one-third (14 l) will be extracellular (ECF).

The extracellular fluid is subdivided into plasma (3 l), interstitial fluid (ISF — an aquatic habitat for the cells, about 10 l) and transcellular fluids (CSF, ocular, peritoneal and synovial fluids, about 1 l).

The osmolalities of the ICF and the ECF are similar although the main cation in the ECF is sodium, whereas in the ICF it is potassium.

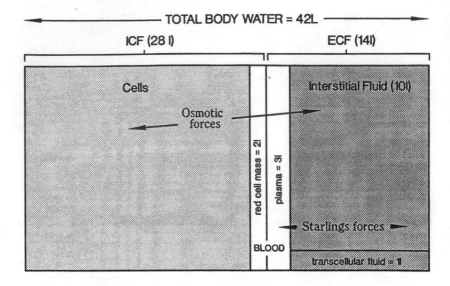

Figure 2.1. Distribution of fluids within the body spaces.

Fluid distribution between the ECF and the ICF is governed only by changes in the osmotic pressure (the ability to attract water). This means that if isotonic fluid (the same osmolality as plasma) is administered into the plasma, it will not enter the ICF, since there is no difference in the osmolality. Fluid distribution between the plasma and the ISF is only governed by Starlings forces (i.e. hydrostatic pressure versus oncotic pressures), and so this fluid would increase the hydrostatic pressure and dilute the oncotic pressure in the plasma until the fluid was evenly distributed throughout the ECF.

TYPES OF FLUID

Crystalloids are essentially electrolytes in water, and because they have no large molecules (and thus have no oncotic pressure), they are easily distributed to the extracellular spaces and are therefore used as maintenance fluids. Examples are normal saline, which is isotonic, and 5% dextrose, which is hypotonic. There is also a solution called Hartmans, which contains lactate, potassium and calcium in addition to sodium chloride, and is therefore meant to be more "physiological".

Colloids contain larger molecules which stay in the circulation for longer and can increase the oncotic pressure and thus may draw fluid back into the circulation. They are good for maintaining the blood pressure; unfortunately they do not have oxygen-carrying capacity. Examples of such are Haemaccel, which contains gelatin, and Dextran, which is a solution of high molecular weight dextrose.

Why is this important? Well, if for example one gave a litre of isotonic saline intravenously, it would initally only be distributed into the ECF (which includes the plasma). As plasma is only 3 l and the whole ECF is 14 l, only 3/14 or 214 ml would remain in the plasma (the distribution takes minutes). In contrast, a litre of 5% dextrose given intravenously which is hypotonic (would initially dilute the ECF relative to the ICF) would be equally distributed throughout the body, and so 3/42 of a litre or 70 ml would remain in the plasma. However, 500 ml of a colloid given intravenously would expand the plasma by 500 ml and, because there is no change in osmotic pressure, will not initially distribute into the cells (ICF). It is clear that different situations require different types of fluid replacement, and you can see why crystalloid preparations are of little use in acute blood loss when colloids or blood may be more appropriate.

THE FLUID BALANCE EQUATION

The simplest way to think about fluid balance is that it is an equilibrium, where input must equal output.

In order to live we must excrete all of our waste products. The main route for this is via the kidneys. The minimal volume of urine we need to produce in order to be healthy is about 1 l a day (0.5–1 ml/kg/h). This is the minimal obligatory volume of urine (MOVU). If less urine than this is produced, the patient is oliguric; and if no urine is produced, anuric.

At rest we also make insensible water losses (fluid losses that we are unaware of) from the lungs and in faeces which amount to about 500 ml, and from the skin by sweating, which is also about 500 ml.

The minimal fluid replacement is therefore about 1.5–2 l. However, this would be a healthy adult lying in bed; if we got up and moved around, then we would have greater requirements. Therefore, we usually reckon that the average adult will require about 3 l in a day.

As well as water, we also lose about 60 mM potassium and 100 mM sodium per day; these salts will also need replacing.

In the normal person large amounts of fluid are recycled in the body and therefore play a part in the equilibrium. These include gastric juice (3–4 l), bile (about 1 l), and intestinal secretions (succus entericus, about 3–4 l). This enteric recycling accounts for about 8 l/day and is mostly reabsorbed further down the GI tract.

It is common sense that we must replace these losses of fluids and electrolytes if we are to remain in equilibrium. This is usually achieved by our daily dietary intake of food and drink, although a small proportion of water is derived as a by-product of metabolism.

When patients come to hospital they may be unable to have sufficient oral intake. This may be because they are "nil by mouth" (perioperatively

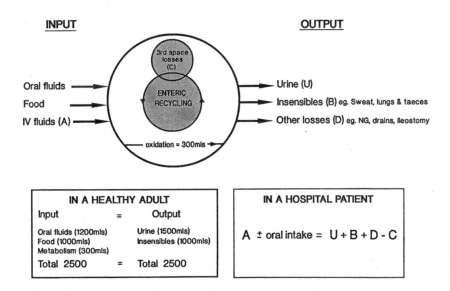

Figure 2.2. The balance between fluid input and fluid output.

or through illness) or they may be vomiting. These patients will require intravenous fluids, with any of the available crystalloid preparations.

As highlighted above, the average adult will need about 3 l a day. This amount of dextrose saline would do (each litre bag contains 30 mM of sodium). Another method would be to give 1 l normal saline (containing 150 mM sodium) and 2 l of 5% dextrose. The dextrose is quickly metabolised, leaving water. In either of these two methods you have replaced 3 l of water with either 90 or 150 mM of sodium. If you add 20 mM of potassium to each litre bag (some bags come with this already added), then you will also replace the necessary 60 mM of potassium. If you request each bag to run over eight hours, then the 3 l will last the full day. If you give nothing but dextrose saline over a period of a few days, the patient may become hyponatraemic.

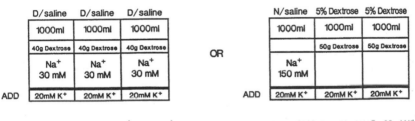

Figure 2.3. Typical daily requirement of intravenous fluids; two alternative regimens.

This is the standard regimen given to most normal adults; there are, however, many exceptions to the rule. These are as follows:

(1) *The Postoperative Period*

The metabolic response to the stresses of surgery involves a rise in various hormones, such as circulating catecholamines, ADH, and through stimulation of the hypothalamo-pituitary-adrenal axis, secretion of cortisol and aldosterone. The overall result of these is the renal conservation of salt and water, with somewhat increased losses of potassium and hydrogen ions. These effects usually last for about 24–48 h.

Despite the high potassium losses in the urine, the serum potassium is usually maintained due to large intracellular stores. One may even see a transient rise in plasma potassium, through release of cellular contents by damaged tissues. Therefore, unless serum potassium levels are very low, it is probably best to avoid potassium supplements in the first day or two postoperatively.

As water is being retained it is usual to reduce the fluid replacements to about 2 l in the first day postop, especially in patients prone to heart failure.

Remember that the patient going to the theatre is likely to have been starved for several hours beforehand and may not have been given any fluids intraoperatively or whilst in recovery. This patient will probably need extra fluids to maintain his fluid balance equilibrium. It is easy to see why one cannot rely on standard regimens when calculating how much fluid to give someone. Urine output is the best indicator, aiming for greater than 50 ml/h. Young fit adults can usually tolerate excess fluids, so as long as the urine output is satisfactory you are probably doing okay. The minimum urine output is about 30 ml/h (remember MOVU). Obviously the urea and electrolytes (U & E's) should be checked, to help assess renal function.

(2) *Third Space Losses*

As mentioned before, about 8 l of secretions per day are reabsorbed in the bowel. If the patient has undergone abdominal surgery he is likely to have a transient ileus postoperatively, where the bowel temporarily stops working. In such patients this is usually due to mechanical handling of the bowel, although any patient can suffer a transient ileus, often due to an electrolyte disturbance or even the effects of anaesthesia.

When an ileus is present, the fluid secreted into the bowel simply lies there, and is not reabsorbed completely. These "third space" losses mean that the patient effectively has a reduced volume of the ECF, and hence is fluid-depleted.

This complicates the management of such patients, as extra fluid needs to be given to allow for the third space losses. Unfortunately you will not know how much extra fluid is needed and so must rely on urine output as an indicator. You will usually notice a sudden diuresis on day 2 or 3 postop. This is explained by recovery of the ileus and reabsorption of the fluids from the bowel.

Similarly, in pancreatitis, patients can lose several litres of fluids rich in electrolytes and plasma proteins into the peritoneal cavity. Really the only way to effectively gauge these losses is by vigorous replacement to maintain their urine output and correcting any electrolyte disturbances according to daily U & Es.

If after two days 10 l have been put in with only 3 l of urine produced, one can assume that about 5 or 6 l have been sequestered into the peritoneal cavity (after subtracting insensible losses).

(3) *Other Losses*

If a patient has a nasogastric tube or a wound drain or is draining via a fistula, these losses need to be calculated daily and replaced (usually as normal saline) in addition to the standard losses.

Ileostomy patients can have huge losses, especially several days postoperatively. It is advisable to assess the ileostomy output at least twice daily, replacing these fluids and electrolytes appropriately to prevent acute dehydration.

Patients with pyrexia require more fluids. One can lose 3 l, maybe more, in certain circumstances. A rough estimate is to increase the fluid replacement by 10% for each degree of fever.

Similarly, losses through vomiting or diarrhoea need replacing; remember that large-intestinal juices contain high concentrations of potassium. Similarly, gastric juice contains lots of hydrogen ions.

(4) *Heart or Liver Failure*

Because the renin–angiotensin system is already working overtime, conserving sodium, you should avoid giving fluids which contain sodium. Use only 5% dextrose in these patients.

In heart failure, the patient is fluid-overloaded, the usual cause in surgical patients being poor management of the fluid balance by the doctor. If you look at the fluid balance charts you will probably see a positive balance over the previous few days. Therefore, you will need to reduce their input, maybe even stop the fluids and consider diuretics. Obviously, you should examine the patient regularly, measuring their JVP, listening to their chest and watching for oedema. Very sick patients on the ward usually will have a CVP line, and this makes the assessment of these patients easier. You should ask the nursing staff to chart the patient's weight daily, as this will help in monitoring progress.

(5) *Acute Renal Failure*
This can be prerenal (hypovolaemia), renal (acute tubular necrosis) or postrenal (e.g. a blocked catheter).

After an operation both pre- and postrenal causes are the commonest, and so should be looked for and treated first. If the patient is fluid-depleted, this may respond simply by correcting the dehydration. Look over the fluid balance charts from the previous days (is this patient in negative fluid balance?). If you think that a renal cause is likely you should avoid potassium loads, stop any drugs that may affect renal function (such as NSAIDS, ACE inhibitors, etc.) and involve the renal team in the management early. Usually they advise replacing the previous days' output plus 500 ml to cover insensible losses. Alternatively one could measure hourly urine output and replace 100% of this every hour.

In summary, input should equal output unless the above exceptions apply. Look over the fluid balance charts (remember, however, that in practice these are often inaccurate) and the daily weight charts. Assess the patient's state of hydration (skin turgor, etc.), look at his blood results for renal function and haematocrit, and do not forget the temperature, both the patient's and the room.

We have deliberately gone into a lot of details on this subject, perhaps more than you need to know to pass finals. This is because it is not really a topic that one can waffle about in the viva — either you understand the principles or you do not.

NUTRITION

Patients who are malnourished suffer with other complications, such as delayed wound healing, muscle weakness and an increased tendency to infection. There is evidence that patients with poor nourishment prior to surgery will benefit from preoperative supplementation, and thus do better after their operation. However, this intervention must be for a reasonable period of time (more than 10 days), in order to be of significant benefit.

There are lots of reasons why hospital patients become poorly nourished. They may be related to the illness itself leading to a decreased appetite, increased needs or impaired digestion, etc., or they may be related to being in hospital; patients being rushed off for an X-ray or ultrasound at 12 p.m., or being nil by mouth. Then there is the much-joked-about-but-oh-so-true dislike of hospital foods, and for certain ethnic minorities the English diet may be alien and unpalatable.

If oral intake is not anticipated within 7–10 days after surgery, then nutritional support is indicated (perhaps 5 days in a previously malnourished patient). The indication for preoperative nutritional support is when a patient is severely malnourished (greater than 10% weight loss).

Nutritional support can vary from mere supplementation of vitamins, or protein in a high protein diet, to a complete replacement of all essential foodstuffs. We will cover only the latter.

Enteral vs. Parenteral Nutrition

Enteral diets are those given via the gut, and they include oral intake. Obviously the ideal situation is one where the patient takes in all the required nutrition orally; if this is not possible then *enteral feeding* involves passing the food into the gut, allowing it to be absorbed normally, either through a nasogastric tube or, if required for longer periods, via a gastrostomy or jejenostomy. The commonest indication for this is where there is a problem with swallowing, such as after a stroke or with oesophageal obstruction.

Parenteral nutrition involves giving a specialised feed directly into the patient's bloodstream, therefore bypassing the gut. It could be given through a simple venflon, but because the feed has a high osmolality and is toxic to veins it really needs to be given via a small cannulae into a large vein with a high rate of blood flow. Hence a CVP line is usually used. For a longer term a Hickman line is used, which is a modified CVP line usually tunneled under the skin to make it more secure and has a Dacron cuff to prevent infection from entering.

Unfortunately, parenteral feeding has some complications, including an increased risk of infection.

- It is not uncommon for a house officer to get called to see a patient with parenteral feeding who has recently spiked a temperature. Obviously your management would be as for any pyrexia (see p. 35); however, if you suspect that the feed is the likely source of the infection, the correct thing to do is to stop the feed. If indeed this is the cause, then the temperature usually settles quickly, despite the fact that the CVP line is still *in situ* and may be infected. It appears that the running feed may be responsible for introducing the bugs from the infected line into the bloodstream. The CVP line will ultimately need to be removed and replaced.
- Another complication of parenteral feeding is villous atrophy in the gut. Since the gut luminal cells (enterocytes) derive their nutrition from the lumen, long periods of rest can lead to atrophy. This makes the gut wall more permeable to bacterial flora and there is evidence that this can increase the risk of "translocation" of bacteria into the bloodstream.
- Electrolyte imbalances are likely and therefore the urea and electrolytes should be checked daily and adjusted accordingly. Hyperglycaemia is another problem and the patient may need to be given insulin temporarily whilst on TPN. Other disturbances of liver function are common (possibly because of fatty infiltration of the liver) and a cholestatic picture may be seen with raised alkaline phosphatase, and hence LFTs should be measured every few days.

The take-home message must be that parenteral feeding should be reserved for patients in whom enteral feeding is impossible, such as patients with short gut syndrome, where large pieces of their gut have been surgically removed. Otherwise enteral feeding should be your first choice.

Requirements

(1) **Water**. See section on fluid balance; roughly 2–3 l per day.
(2) **Energy**. About 1800 calories per day. This is given as a mixture of carbohydrate and fats. Roughly in a ratio of two-thirds to one-third respectively (but can be up to 50–50).
(3) **Nitrogen**. About 14 g per day in protein, but the requirement may change (8–20 g/day) according to the metabolic state.
(4) **Vitamins**. The fat-soluble vitamins are stored and so the levels are carefully adjusted to avoid overdosage. Water-soluble vitamins being excreted are therefore given more generously.
(5) **Minerals**. Sodium, potassium, calcium, magnesium, phosphate, etc.
(6) **Trace elements**. Zinc, copper, iron, selenium, iodide, etc.

The decision about whether to start nutrition is made by the surgeon; however, the important people in the actual implementation of this are the pharmacist, who makes up the feed, and the nurses, who actually give it. Nowadays the feeds are usually made up into one complete sterile 3 l bag (even if it contains only 2 l) in the pharmacy department according to the specific requirements of the individual, hopefully with the dietician's advice. The nursing staff connect it to the patient, and this is the most important step as this is when infection is likely to occur, and hence it should be a sterile procedure.

Monitoring assessment of nutritional status is best done on a clinical basis. The patient's appearance and weight are the best indicators. Other anthropometric measurements, such as skin fold thickness, are not ideal but may be of benefit in monitoring progress.

Daily measurement of albumin is pointless, since its half-life is long (about 21 days) and its level can be altered for many other reasons, although it is helpful in long term monitoring.

Other biochemical tests are available, such as transferrin, which is better than albumin in the short term. But probably the best day-to-day biochemical measurement is prealbumin (a liver protein), which is a good marker of nutritional status. Obviously, electrolytes should be measured daily and LFTs should be checked every few days.

Finally, of much amusement on ward rounds are the other markers of nutrition, such as grip strength and stool length — but as to who does these, let alone how, I leave to your imagination.

3

PRE- AND POSTOPERATIVE MANAGEMENT

When you are a houseman your role preoperatively will be to clerk the patients and prepare them for the theatre or their investigations and to organize the theatre lists.

A clerking consists of the history of the presenting complaint, past medical history, drug history, family history and social history. You should then examine the patient fully, looking first at his general health and whether he is fit enough for the operation, and if not you should be thinking of ways to optimize his health, such as using preoperative nebulizers for an asthmatic. The clerking also allows other problems to be picked up. If, when the patient arrives on the ward, you feel that the diagnosis made in the out-patient clinic has changed, you should inform a senior colleague before the operation is booked. For example, if a patient is due for an excisional biopsy of a lymph node that has completely disappeared when you see him, then you should inform your consultant, so that the operation can be cancelled.

The appropriate investigations should have been performed before surgery and you may be asked about this in your viva. For example, before a laparascopic cholecystectomy can be performed the patient should have had an ultrasound to confirm the presence of gallstones, and a set of liver function tests.

The houseman discusses with the operating surgeon the order in which they would like to have the patients on the list. Usually children are placed first on the list, as this is nicer for the child and the parents; also they find it hard to go without food for long periods. If special equipment is needed in the theatre, such as the image intensifier for

X-rays or laparascopic equipment, then these can be discussed with the theatre staff (and radiographers) the day beforehand.

Specialist nurses such as the breast care nurse or stoma nurse should be involved preoperatively in all appropriate cases. For example, a patient who may need a colostomy or ileostomy should be seen by the stoma nurse several days before the operation. This is, firstly, to educate the patient and answer his questions and worries, and secondly, to mark the site where the stoma will be (with the patient standing).

Many patients have problems other than the one that is to be operated on. These may be social, such as the need for a social-work or occupational-therapy referral. The patients may have intercurrent medical problems such as diabetes, hypertension or COAD. They may also be on drugs such as steroids or anticoagulants. When clerking the patient you should be looking out for these, and if you think they may affect the operation, then you should inform the anaesthetist or the consultant in charge of the patient.

As a housemen the tests you need to consider preoperatively are blood tests such as a full blood count, a sickle screen if at risk, and either a group and save or cross-match. You should X-match any patient at risk of blood loss extensive enough to need replacing — for example, the anticipated blood loss from an anterior resection is about two units, but to be safe we usually X-match four units. The blood is kept in the refrigerator ready for use. If it is not used it goes back to the blood bank and is stored.

A young healthy person in general requires no preoperative investigations, but if at all unsure then the houseman should discuss with the anaesthetist what they would like performed (for example, some anaesthetists like to have a recent full blood count on all females of childbearing age). If the patient is hypertensive or on diuretics then a U & E's (urea, creatinine and electrolytes) to assess renal function must be performed. An ECG is necessary on anyone who is hypertensive or has a history of heart disease, and a chest X-ray on anyone with respiratory diseases, including a personal or family history of TB. In most hospitals the requirement is to order an ECG and CXR as a baseline on the elderly (aged over 60), but check the policy in your hospital.

The management of medical problems in surgical patients is essentially the same as that you read about in medical textbooks. We will, however, cover just a few topics:

DIABETES

Diabetics have an increased incidence of perioperative complications. The stress of surgery can lead to an increased production of catabolic hormones, such as glucagon and catecholamines, which antagonize the action of insulin, making control more difficult, especially as the patient will also be nil by mouth. These patients are at an increased risk of infection (wound, chest, IV access sites and urine), peripheral vascular disease, pressure sores and ischaemic heart disease.

The aim is to maintain the patient's blood sugar level between 5 and 9 mmol/l. Preoperatively you should dipstick the urine to check for protein, send off a laboratory glucose, check the electrolytes and creatinine, and order an ECG.

Management depends on whether the patient is insulin- dependent or not.

Insulin-dependent diabetics. For anything other than minor surgery it is probably best to put these patients on an insulin sliding scale to establish good control. This means they are on a drip of dextrose or dextrose saline (as they are not eating), together with a continuous infusion of fast-acting insulin. The rate of infusion of insulin will depend on their blood sugar level, which can be monitored by hourly BM stix (a finger prick testing stick specific for glucose). If the BM is low the infusion is decreased or stopped, and if the BM is high the insulin rate can be increased to bring the sugar level down. It is of vital importance that you add potassium to each bag of fluids you give, since the insulin causes cellular uptake of potassium and can lead to hypokalaemia. The sliding scales differ in different hospitals and you should try and get hold of a sliding scale from the protocol at your hospital. This is one example:

BM (mM/L)		0–4	4–8	8–12	12–16	> 16
Rate of insulin per hour (units/h)		0.5	1.0	2.0	4.0	6.0

Diabetics controlled with oral hypoglycaemics. Long-acting oral hypoglycaemics such as metformin should be changed to a short-acting sulphonylurea (e.g. Gliclazide) a few days before the operation. Ask the diabetic team for advice. On the morning of the operation do not give the dose of the sulphonylurea. This can be resumed once the patient starts eating postoperatively. The BMs can be measured, and if very high the blood sugar can be brought down by small doses of subcutaneous soluble insulin (e.g. 6 units of actrapid). If this fails to control the diabetes successfully or if it is a major operation, then you can simply convert them to a sliding scale as above. Diabetics should really go first on the list, as the starting time is predictable and this allows you to manage the sugar levels better.

Diabetics controlled by diet alone rarely need any special measures. Remember that provided they have not been given any insulin or oral hypoglycaemics they cannot become hypoglycaemic; if anything their sugar level will be high. A BM stix will tell you where you stand if you are worried. If you find their control is poor then you should refer the patients back to their diabetologist.

STEROIDS

Patients on steroids are liable to impaired healing and postoperative infections. Also, long term corticosteroids can lead to adrenal insufficiency. The adrenals are unable secrete the increased glucocorticoids necessary in response to the stresses of surgery. This can lead to an Addisonian crisis, where the patient becomes shocked. Patients who have been on long term oral steroids should therefore be covered with perioperative steroids. We usually give intravenous hydrocortisone before and after the operation until the patient can resume their oral intake.

CHRONIC OBSTRUCTIVE AIRWAY DISEASE (COAD/COPD)

Surgery and anaesthesia predispose patients to basal lung collapse (atelectasis), aspiration pneumonitis and chest infection. This is especially true of operations to the abdomen, since the patients are in pain and therefore do not cough up the secretions in their lungs. Any pre-existing respiratory disease, such as COAD, increases the risk of chest complications, as do smoking, obesity and old age.

Preoperatively therefore you should arrange for a chest X-ray and lung function tests in any patient with pre-existing chronic airways disease. You should also do a baseline blood gas analysis if hypoxia or carbon dioxide retention is anticipated.

You can assess the degree of reversibility of the airway disease by measuring peak flows before and after bronchodilators given by nebulizer. If there is a degree of reversibility the prescription of nebulizers may help optimize lung function.

Physiotherapy is the most important modality in these patients. Preoperative breathing exercises and advice help to prevent a chest infection, and early postoperative physiotherapy to help remove airway secretions is vital, especially in abdominal operations. Smokers should be encouraged to stop smoking at least four weeks prior to elective surgery.

DEEP VEIN THROMBOSIS (DVT)

All surgical patients are at risk of DVT. In some hospitals prophylaxis with subcutaneous heparin injections (5000 units two to three times a day) and thromboembolic deterrent (TED) stockings is given to all surgical patients, whereas other hospitals only give this to patients at medium-to-high risk of DVT. Risk factors include previous DVT or pulmonary embolus, long periods of immobility, pelvic or hip operations, obesity, cancer, use of the oral contraceptive pill, etc. Again check your hospital's protocol. Newer methods of prophylaxis include intermittent limb compression, where an inflatable device is wrapped around the legs and periodically blown up, from the distal to the proximal end, encouraging venous return. Also available is low molecular weight heparin (LMW), which is thought to work on the antiplatelet factor antithrombin III and therefore has little effect on the intrinsic clotting cascade and so in normal prophylactic doses does not require monitoring; it is longer-acting and thus only needs to be given once daily. LMW heparin is as effective as unfractionated heparins.

ANTIBIOTICS

Some operations carry an increased risk of infective complications. We therefore give prophylactic antibiotics to anyone at a significant risk of developing an infection. This may be because of factors related to the type of operation, or because of factors related to the patient. Contaminated operations, such as those where the bowel contents can leak out, carry a high risk of infection, as do operations where a prosthetic implant is used (e.g. joint replacement), and antibiotics should always be given in these cases. An example of a patient-related factor is mitral valve disease and the subsequent risk of developing endocarditis.

We usually give prophylactic antibiotics intravenously at induction, so that blood levels are high during the operation, followed by two subsequent doses postoperatively. If a tourniquet is being used, then the antibiotics must be given before the tourniquet is inflated.

You should have a rough idea of which organisms are likely to be responsible for the infection and which antibiotics should therefore be used. A common question concerns MRSA (methicillin-resistant *Staphylococcus aureus*), which is an increasing problem in many hospitals.

Operations Involving the Bowel

Organisms. Mainly gram −ve bacilli, i.e. *coliforms*, but also faecal *anaerobes* (bacteroides) and *Staphylococcus aureus* from the skin. In the gut there is also *Enterococcus faecalis* (also known as *strep faecalis*), but this causes infection less commonly. In bile, the majority of infections are with gut bacteria, such as *E. coli*, and rarely *pseudomonas*, which is more difficult to treat.

Prophylaxis. We tend to use a cephalosporin to cover the gram –ve organisms together with metronidazole to cover anaerobes. If you are concerned about strep faecalis you should add amoxycillin, as the cephalosporins do not cover this well.

For operations on the biliary tree, such as a laparascopic cholecystectomy, you could either use the same regimen as above or just use a cephalosporin alone, as most infections are with gram –ve bacilli (mainly *E. coli*). One dose at induction is sufficient. For improved biliary penetration such as before and after an ERCP or for ascending cholangitis, a broad spectrum β-lactam such as pipericillin is often used. This also covers for pseudomonas.

Operations Involving Prosthetic Implants

Organisms. Skin organisms are usually responsible. *Staphylococcus aureus* is the commonest pathogen, but also *Staphylococcus epidermidis* tends to colonize the newer plastic prostheses. Rarely, coliforms are responsible.

Prophylaxis. Either a broad spectrum cephalosporin or flucloxacillin. Orthopaedic operations involving metalwork require a dose of intravenous antibiotics (usually a cephalosporin) at induction and for about 24 h postoperatively. Similarly, valve replacements are usually given flucloxacillin (or a cephalosporin) and gentamycin. If MRSA is a particular worry, then vancomycin may be used.

Remember that if ischaemic or necrotic tissue is involved then spores of clostridium tetani may cause gas gangrene. Benzylpenicillin, to which the organism is highly susceptible, is the prophylaxis (and treatment) of choice against this (this includes penetrating wounds and compound fractures).

If you were asked to write an essay on preoperative management, you might find it useful to remember the list ABCD LMNOP's:

A — Antibiotics/Anaesthetist
B — Bloods (incl. X-match)/Bowel preparation
C — Consent/CXR
D — Drug chart/DVT prophylaxis
E — ECG
F — Fluids (esp. if NBM or if the patient is vomiting)
L — List (put in the theatre list)/Lung function tests
M — Mark the area or limb (should be done by the operating surgeon)
N — Notes filed correctly
O — Operating theatre staff (e.g. special equipment/radiology)
P — Physiotherapy
S — Specialist nurses (e.g. breast care or stoma care nurses).

POSTOPERATIVELY

The role of the houseman postoperatively is to check that the patient has recovered from the anaesthetic, look at their observation charts and check their fluid balance. The operation note should have a section on specific postoperative management written by the surgeon, and is a guide that should be followed. For example, following a vascular graft operation — say, to the leg — you should always check the pulses, capillary refill and toe movement in the involved leg to ensure that the graft has not blocked off.

A common question for finals concerns talking about complications of operations.

Complications

All operations carry a risk of complications. These can be divided into *general* and *specific*. General complications include those pertaining to the anaesthesia itself and those that can occur after any operation, such as a chest infection or DVT. Specific complications are those that occur because of the individual operation itself, such as cutting a nerve.

You should subdivide this classification into complications that occur *immediately*, within the first 24 h; *early*, within the first week or so; *late postoperative*, occurring within the first month or so; and *long term*.

General immediate complications include those due to the anaesthetic, such as direct trauma to the mouth when intubating and reactions to the anaesthetic (inherited disorders or idiosyncratic reactions). Early complications include chest infections, urinary retention or infections, deep vein thrombosis, bed sores, etc.

Specific complications depend on the nature of the operation. In this section haemorrhage and wound infection are important.

Haemorrhage

This can be divided into primary, reactionary and secondary haemorrhage.

Primary haemorrhage occurs during the operation, when a vessel is cut. Reactionary haemorrhage is when at the end of the operation the wound looks dry, but when the patient's blood pressure and cardiac output come up to normal levels it begins to bleed, presumably from vessels that were not properly ligated during the operation. Secondary haemorrhage, occurring several days after the operation, is usually attributed to infection that erodes through a vessel.

Wound Infections

These are most commonly caused by *Staphylococcus aureus*, although coliforms such as *E. coli* are also important. Wound infection is more likely if:

- The operation is dirty (e.g. abdominal).
- The duration of the operation is long (greater than 2 h).
- The patient is more susceptible (e.g. old age, immunosuppression, diabetes).

Minor wound infections, with a little redness and slight discharge, are relatively common and usually need just simple measures, such as regular wound dressing and perhaps antibiotics. More severe infections, common after abdominal operations, usually occur in the first week or so. The wound looks inflamed, and there may be cellulitis, discharge or localised abscess formation. The wound should be swabbed and maybe antibiotics started, but the only correct treatment for an abscess is drainage. This may mean simply removing a few of the surgical clips, and probing the wound, allowing the pus to discharge, or a further surgical procedure to open up the wound. The wound is then left to heal by secondary intention (i.e. to heal itself from within, with no further suturing).

Wound Dehiscence

This is an uncommon problem. It is usually due to an inadequate repair of the tissues (but infection, poor blood supply, malnutrition and steroids may all play a part in poor wound healing). Dehiscence usually occurs about a week after the operation. A warning sign is a sero-sanguinous

	Specific	General
Immediate (within 24 h)	Haemorrhage Damage to adjacent structures	Reaction to anaesthesia Asphyxia
Early (1st week or so)	Paralytic ileus Anastomotic leak Infection — wound — deep collection	Chest infection UTI Pulmonary embolus DVT Bed sores
Late (1st month)	Inability to eat normal size meals Dumping syndrome Steatorrhoea/diarrhoea Weight loss (combination of above)	Consequences of complications either specific or general in early post-operative period
Long term	Anaemia — Pernicious — Iron-deficient Osteoporosis Recurrence of ulcer Malignancy	

discharge from the wound a few days before. The wound suddenly bursts open and in a laparotomy the bowel protrudes outwards and is extremely alarming for the patient and nursing staff. Sterile soaked swabs should be placed over the wound and the patient taken back to the theatre for repair.

An example of general and specific complications pertaining to a gastrectomy is outlined below. The general section will be the same for all operations. Try and draw up a list of the specific complications for other common procedures, such as operations on the colon, thyroid and breast. For further elaboration see the chapter on stomach operations.

The commonest problems that a housemen will get called to the wards for are to write up fluids or to see a postoperative pyrexia or poor urine output.

POSTOPERATIVE PYREXIA

A small rise in temperature is common postoperatively. If the temperature spikes above 38° or persists, then you should consider and look for the 7 C's as potential causes. This is a common viva question.

- *Chest* — chest infection
- *Catheter* — UTI
- *CVP line* — infected
- *Cannula* — superficial thrombophlebitis (remove cannula)
- *Cut* — wound infection
- *Collection* — subphrenic or pelvic abscess (may indicate a failure of anastomosis)
- *Calves* — DVT (rumbling pyrexia in second postoperative week)

A *chest infection* is very common postop, especially in patients who smoke or have pre-existing poor respiratory function. The mucus secretions are not cleared; these then clog up the smaller bronchi, which leads to collapse of the air spaces distal to the blockage (atelectasis). Inhaled organisms then infect the collapsed segments. Thoracic and upper abdominal incisions cause pain and stop the patients from coughing up the secretions, and they are much more likely to have basal atelectasis and develop chest infections. These patients should therefore be given adequate analgesia, have vigorous physiotherapy, and be encouraged to cough up the phlegm (whilst holding their wounds — applicable for chest and abdominal wounds).

A deep collection, such as a *subphrenic or pelvic abscess*, can occur after the patient has had generalized peritonitis. The patient usually presents with general malaise, nausea, pain (a subphrenic abscess may also cause pain felt in the shoulder tip), a swinging pyrexia and localized peritonitis. A pelvic abscess often occurs 4–10 days postop, whereas a subphrenic abscess usually occurs a bit later, 7–21 days postop. Clinically the patient appears to be recovering well, but then develops a fever and starts to feel unwell. The white cell count may be raised and a collection is identified on ultrasound or CT. Treatment is by drainage, either percutaneously under ultrasound or CT guidance, or by an open procedure. A drain is usually left *in situ*.

A small anastomotic leak usually causes a localized abscess which becomes sealed off by the omentum and the bowel. Clinically the patient is slow to recover, but usually improves with intravenous antibiotics and fluids and delayed return to food. A larger anastomotic breakdown causes the patient to be very unwell, with anything from local peritonitis through to a rigid abdomen and septicaemia. The abscess needs to be drained, the peritoneal cavity washed out, and the two ends of the failed anastomosis can be brought out as temporary stomas.

A diagnosis of DVT and pulmonary embolus in the first instance is essentially a clinical one, as treatment is usually instituted before definitive diagnosis is made. A pulmonary embolus (PE) usually presents with pleuritic chest pain (stabbing and worse on inspiration). The textbooks tend to describe the findings in a large PE, although more commonly in the smaller PE's the findings are less impressive and the patient may even be asymptomatic. The patient is usually tachycardic, maybe with a low grade fever and maybe tachypnoeic, but not much else. The ECG usually shows sinus tachycardia (the classic S1Q3T3, which most students know about, occurs when there is a large amount of right heart strain, in a large PE, and is rarely seen). The CXR is usually unhelpful but may show a small area of linear atelectasis. Blood gas analysis is essential and you would expect to find a low PO2 (due to ventilation/perfusion mismatches) and a low PCO_2 due to hyperventilation. Examination of the calves may or may not reveal evidence of a DVT. If a DVT or PE is suspected, we usually start a heparin infusion before we investigate. To diagnose a DVT you can use duplex ultrasound (or a venogram) and to diagnose a PE you can request a ventilation–perfusion scan (or pulmonary venography).

Other less common causes for a fever include infective diarrhoeas, drug reactions and blood transfusion reactions.

If faced with a patient with a pyrexia you would obviously find out a little history and examine the patient properly. In a viva situation you could say to the examiner, "I would listen to the chest, examine the abdomen, check the cannula sites, inspect the wound, etc... My investigations would depend on my clinical findings but may involve sending a urine specimen, a full blood count and blood cultures, sending wound swabs or the tip of the central line for culture, etc."

DRAINS

Collections within a wound which often contain blood are the perfect medium for colonization of bacteria and hence infection; therefore a drain is used to remove any anticipated collections within a wound. They are not substitutes for adequate haemostasis at the time of the operation. Drains can be closed or open.

Closed drainage includes suction drainage (i.e. Redivac) and means that the collection is attracted into a bottle usually by suction. This reduces the risk of infection and is used for large spaces or cavities, such as after a mastectomy or joint replacement. Drains are usually removed as soon as possible (usually 24–48 h) or as soon as the losses begin to tail off. They should not usually be left in for more than 5 days as they can actually introduce infection.

Open drainage, such as a piece of corrugated tubing with one end in the wound and the other in a dressing, allows small losses to escape from the wound. This is often employed in established abscesses after incision and drainage to allow any remaining collection a passage out of the wound. Some surgeons like to withdraw this type of drain in stages to allow the track to collapse behind it.

Other drains commonly asked about in finals include chest drains, T-tubes and percutaneous nephrostomies (see relevant sections).

POSTOPERATIVE POOR URINE OUTPUT

A common viva question. The cause can be prerenal, renal or postrenal. The commonest causes of failure to pass urine postoperatively are postrenal.

Postrenal problems (commoner in males) include obstruction caused by a large prostate or a blocked catheter. Firstly the patient may find it difficult to initiate micturition; this may be due to anticholinergic drugs given with the anaesthetic, perhaps because of pain (for example after a hernia repair), or the patient may simply be inhibited because of strange surroundings or a nurse continually asking him if he has passed urine yet. Then the bladder becomes so distended that it fails to function properly. Benign prostatic hypertrophy is an important predisposition and these patients are more likely to go into retention.

Prerenal causes are due to renal hypoperfusion because of either hypovolaemia or heart failure.

Renal causes. Acute renal failure is usually due to acute tubular necrosis.

When a house officer you will commonly be called to see a patient who has failed to pass urine postoperatively. Often this will be a patient you are covering but do not know about, and so you should find out what operation was performed and when. In your history you should search for clues pointing to whether the problem is pre- or postrenal. Ask if there is any pain; an enlarged bladder causes suprapubic pain, although this is difficult to differentiate from pain in an abdominal wound (one exception is when there is an epidural *in situ* and there is no pain). On examination you should look for signs of hypovolaemia (dry mucous membranes, decreased skin turgor, tachycardia, etc.), signs of heart failure (shortness of breath, tachycardia, raised CVP or JVP and bibasillar crepitations, peripheral oedma, etc.). A distended bladder palpable just above the pubis is dull to percussion and usually tender and when touched makes the patient want to pass urine.

If you suspect that the cause is postrenal (distended bladder and discomfort), then the diagnosis is proven by catheterization. A large residual volume of urine should drain (usually about 500 ml or more). You can initially try conservative measures such as analgesia, privacy, siting in a warm bath, etc., but if that fails then catheterization is indicated. If the patient already has a catheter *in situ*, then the catheter should be flushed to ensure it is not blocked. If the urine coming out of the catheter is small amounts of concentrated dark urine, then the cause is likely to be prerenal anyway. You could dipstick it testing for a high specific gravity (> 1020) to prove this.

If clinically the patient does not appear to be in retention, you should check the fluid balance charts. Observe how much fluid has gone in before, during and since the operation and the measured urine output. Remember that a long laparotomy can lead to large losses of fluid by evaporation and this will not be measured on the charts. A urine output of less than about 30 ml per hour is poor (oliguria). Really the patient should be catheterized anyway at this point to measure the hourly urine output. U & E's should be sent; if there is a prerenal cause, the urea will be raised. If from your clinical examination and your assessment of the fluid balance charts you think the patient has a prerenal cause, then you should try a fluid challenge — 250–500 ml of normal saline given as a stat dose (unless you suspect blood loss as the cause, in which case the patient may be shocked and should be given colloids and blood — see section on shock). Then observe the urine output over the next hour. If the urine output picks up, you have shown the patient to be in need of more fluid and the next bag should be speeded up. If the patient has heart failure, the urine output will not pick up and the patient may become a little more breathless and the CVP should rise. If this occurs, a bolus dose of a loop diuretic, such as 40 mg of frusemide, will lead to a diuresis, and a fall in the CVP. If the patient does not have a central line in at this point, you should ask a senior colleague for advice, as a central line is really necessary for knowing exactly what the state of vascular filling is and will help in the management.

Only after you have excluded a postrenal and a prerenal cause can you assume that there may be a renal problem and acute tubular necrosis has occurred. The creatinine will be raised and you should measure the urine and plasma osmolalities. The ratio of urine to plasma osmolality will be less than 1 (as opposed to prerenal oliguria, where the ratio will be > 1). Advice from a renal physician should be sought.

4

TRAUMA, SHOCK,
HEAD INJURIES AND BURNS

ATLS® Used/modified with permission by the American College of Surgeons Committee on Trauma, Advanced Trauma Life Support® Manual 1993, third impression, Chicago.

TRAUMA

Imagine yourself being faced with a multiply injured patient with trauma to the head, chest, abdomen and limbs. Where would you start? What if there were several injured patients, which would take priority?

The Advanced Trauma and Life Support (ATLS®) course was developed following a tragedy. In 1976 an orthopaedic surgeon who was piloting his own plane over rural Nebraska crashed in a cornfield. His wife died instantly and three of his four children sustained critical injuries. They were taken to the nearest medical facility, the surgeon was appalled at the poor quality of care that he and his family received and felt that a system was needed to improve the care of trauma patients.

There is a trimodal distribution of death following injury. The *first peak* occurs at the time of the injury, usually due to severe lacerations of the brain, heart or large blood vessels, and the patient is usually dead before arrival to casualty. Prevention by methods such as seat belts, crash helmets and speed limits is the only effective way of reducing these deaths.

The *second peak* occurs within minutes to hours of the injury. Injuries such as a tension pneumothorax, blood loss and intracranial bleeds account for this peak. These deaths are potentially reversible with immediate medical management.

The *third peak* of deaths occurs several days to weeks after the incident, due to sepsis and multiorgan failure. The care provided during the initial resuscitaion and subsequent period directly affects the outcome of this group.

The concept behind ATLS® is to treat life-threatening injuries first and all other injuries in order of priority, and since a blocked airway kills within seconds this clearly should have first priority; likewise a tension pneumothorax will kill before bleeding from a wound.

The approach is divided into a *primary survey*, where life-threatening injuries are identified; *resuscitation* (in reality the primary survey and resuscitation take place simultaneously, so that when you identify a life-threatening injury, you deal with it immediately); a *secondary survey* (a more thorough head-to-toe examination); and *re-evaluation*. The patient is continuously re-evaluated until he is stable and definitive care for him can be instituted.

Primary Survey

As the patient arrives there is usually some history available — if not from him, then from witnesses or the ambulance crew. His vital signs from when he was first seen by the paramedics till he arrives at the A & E department should be noted.

The primary survey is a rapid evaluation; the mnemonic ABCDE is used to allow one to think in an ordered and prioritized manner.

A — Airway with cervical spine control
B — Breathing and ventilation
C — Circulation with haemorrhage control
D — Disability
E — Exposure and environment

A. *Airway with Cervical Spine Control*

In anyone with an altered level of consciousness or injuries above the clavicles, suspect a cervical spine injury. The patient's head should be supported by a hand on either side to prevent any movement (in-line manual immobilization), and when possible a semirigid collar should be placed on with two sandbags on either side of the head with tape across them.

The airway should be checked to see if it is patent or if there are signs of airway obstruction. Listen for noisy breathing, look for obvious facial trauma, and inspect for foreign bodies by a sweep of your little finger inside the mouth.

B. *Breathing*

Assess the respiratory function. Inspect and palpate for tracheal deviation, expansion of the lungs and for any lacerations, rib fractures or flail segments. A flail chest, commonly asked about in exams, is a segment of the chest wall that, owing to multiple fractures, has no bony continuity with the rest of the thoracic cage. The flail segment moves paradoxically (it moves in on inspiration and out on expiration) with the rest of the chest. The hypoxia that results is usually not due to the flail segment alone but more to the underlying contusion to the lung and hence mismatches between ventilation and perfusion.

C. *Circulation with Haemorrhage Control*

Assess the level of consciousness, pulse, blood pressure, respiratory rate, skin colour and capillary refill time (see page 51). Hypotension following injury must be assumed to be due to hypovolaemia until proved otherwise.

During the primary survey any external severe bleeding points should be controlled by applying a sterile pressure dressing or a pneumatic splint. Tourniquets are usually avoided, as they cause crush injuries and distal ischaemia.

Internal bleeding should be suspected and you should examine systematically for all of the causes, such as an intrathoracic or intra-abdominal bleed or a fractured pelvis and/or femur. A bleed into the cranial cavity will by itself not cause hypovolaemia.

D. *Disability*

This is a rapid neurological evaluation assessing the patient's level of consciousness and the pupil size and response to light.

The pneumonic AVPU is used as a quick assessment of the patient's level of consciousness. If for example the patient responds only to pain, then his AVPU score is P.

A — Alert
V — responds to Verbal stimuli
P — responds to Painful stimuli
U — Unresponsive

The Glasgow Coma Score (GCS) is a more detailed neurological evaluation that can be done in the primary survey although it takes longer, and because the life-threatening A, B and C's take precedence in the primary survey the GCS may be performed in the secondary survey (see section on head injury for details).

A decreased level of consciousness may be due to many factors, including cerebral injury, hypoxia and shock. It may also be secondary to alcohol and drugs, although head injury, hypoxia and shock must be excluded first.

E. *Exposure*

Completely undress the patient (cut off the clothes if necessary), inspect the entire skin surface for evidence of injury, such as bruising, abrasions or lacerations. A log roll should be performed with in-line cervical spine immobilization (i.e. the head is supported and turned in line with the patient to prevent any movement of the cervical spine). The entire vertebral column is palpated down to the coccyx for tenderness and a rectal examination is performed to check for a high-riding prostate (other signs of possible urethral rupture include blood at the urethral meatus or a scrotal haematoma).

During the primary survey a series of X-rays are taken, called the trauma series, which include a C-spine, chest and pelvic X-rays. An ECG is usually taken. A nasogastric tube (beware of a cribiform plate fracture) and urinary catheter (after a rectal examination) should be considered.

RESUSCITATION

As mentioned above, this is carried out simultaneously during the primary survey.

Airway

The airway must be patent and protected in all patients. There are five things you can do; always start with simple measures, such as the chin lift, and progress through the following list until oxygenation is adequate. Apply an oxygen mask with a reservoir (to allow about 85% oxygen).

(1) *Chin lift or jaw thrust.* In the supine position the tongue naturally falls back, obstructing the hypopharynx. These procedures bring the tongue forward, opening up the airway. In the chin lift the chin is grasped between the first finger and the thumb. The chin is then lifted gently and brought anteriorly (being careful not to hyperextend the neck). In the jaw thrust manoeuvre the angles of the mandible are grasped by a hand on each side and the lower jaw is brought forward.
(2) *Guedel airway.* If breathing is still noisy, you can maintain the airway, by inserting an oropharyngeal airway, such as a Guedel airway (an S-shaped plastic tube). The size should correspond to the distance

from the centre of the patient's mouth to the angle of the jaw. It is put in upside down and rotated when it is past the tongue.

(3) *Nasopharyngeal tube.* If the patient is conscious and has a gag reflex, he is unlikely to tolerate an oropharyngeal airway. In this case a nasopharyngeal airway can be tried, as it is better-tolerated and is less likely to induce vomiting, although many conscious patients will not tolerate either and may need to be anaesthetized and intubated.

(4) *Intubation.* This is called a definitive airway, which means a tube is inserted into the trachea with a cuff inflated to prevent aspiration; the whole thing is secured with tape and oxygen is connected. A definitive airway can be an orotracheal tube, a nasotracheal tube or a surgical airway. A definitive airway is needed if the patient is not breathing, is unable to maintain an airway with the above measures, if there is impending airway compromise (as in inhalation injuries), or in a head injury requiring hyperventilation.

As CO_2 is produced in the lungs you can confirm the tube is in the trachea by measuring the end tidal CO_2 tension. If the tube was mistakenly placed into the oesophagus then the CO_2 gas pattern would be absent. Proper placement of the tube is also checked by listening for bilateral air entry (if the tube has entered the right main bronchus then no sounds will be heard on the left).

(5) *Surgical airway.* If you are unable to intubate (for example when there is severe facial trauma, oedema of the glottis, etc.), then a surgical airway is indicated. A tracheostomy is difficult to perform and is time-consuming, and so a needle cricothyroidotomy can be performed [a large calibre cannula is inserted through the cricothyroid membrane into the trachea (feel for Adam's apple, and move you finger downwards till you come to the first gap between the thyroid and cricoid cartilages)]. A needle cricothyroidotomy can be converted to a surgical cricothyroidotomy by widening the incision and placing a cuffed endotracheal tube into the space between the thyroid and cricoid cartilages (remember that a tracheostomy is placed into the trachea at about the level of the second or third tracheal ring and is a much longer

procedure as the thyroid gland has to be divided and is therefore performed in theatre when the patient is stable). Oxygen is then connected to the airway.

Breathing

The word "ATOMIC" has been used to list life-threatening chest injuries, which should be identified in the primary survey:

Airway obstruction
Tension pneumothorax
Open pneumothorax
Massive haemothorax (greater than 1500 ml)
Intercostal disruption (some people modify the mnemonic to ATOM FC, where **F** stands for "Flail chest")
Cardiac tamponade

A *tension pneumothorax* occurs when air enters the pleural space either from outside or from inside the lung. A one-way valve is formed by the pleura, which allows air to enter the pleural space during inspiration, but does not allow it to escape during expiration. The lung collapses, and the mediastinum and the trachea are deviated away from the affected side. The patient becomes very short of breath and cyanotic. The venous return to the heart is impaired and the signs are similar to those of cardiac tamponade (raised JVP and falling BP, but they can be differentiated by listening for breath sounds). The diagnosis is made clinically — a distressed, tachycardic patient with a deviated trachea, hyper-resonance to percussion and absent breath sounds on the affected side. You should never see a chest X-ray on patients with a tension pneumothorax, as they should have been treated immediately before waiting for an X-ray to be taken.

Treatment is by placing a cannula (venflon) into the second intercostal space, mid-clavicular line and hearing a hiss as the air escapes. Once this is performed the tension pneumothorax is converted to a simple pneumothorax and the immediate threat to life is over. A chest drain should be inserted as soon as possible.

Insertion of a Chest Drain

A chest drain is inserted anterior to the mid-axillary line in the fifth intercostal space. If possible (provided no cervical spine injury is suspected) the patient is sat up and the hand is placed behind their neck on the affected side to expose the field and open up the intercostal space. Otherwise the procedure is performed with the patient supine. The area is prepared with betadine and draped. Some anaesthetic is infiltrated to the skin, subcutaneous tissues and down to the pleura. A 2 cm transverse incision is made in the fifth intercostal space (aiming above the rib as the intercostal bundle sits in the groove just below the rib). Blunt dissection is then performed down to the pleura. A pair of forceps is pushed through the pleura into the pleural space. A finger is swept around to free any adhesions and create the space for the tube. A chest tube is inserted using a pair of forceps, usually French gauge 24–28 (if a haemo-pneumothorax exists a larger tube size, Fr. 38, is usually used). The drain is fixed with a stitch and a purse-string or mattress suture is placed in the wound (to allow it to be closed when the drain is removed). The chest drain is connected to an underwater seal (this allows air to escape during expiration, but no air to enter). Ensure that the underwater seal is below the patient, otherwise the water will enter the chest (if you are ever asked to check if a chest drain is blocked, ask the patient to cough; you should see bubbles escaping if it is patent). Re-X-ray the patient after the procedure.

In an open pneumothorax, if the opening is approximately two-thirds of the diameter of the trachea, then air passes through the wound in preference to the airway during inspiration (taking the route of least resistance). This is also called a "sucking chest wound". Close the wound with a sterile dressing taped on three sides to form a flap valve.

Circulation (see page 51)

Two large bore cannulae should be inserted, one into each antecubital fossa of all patients exposed to major trauma. Blood should be taken for a cross-match, a full blood count, and urea and electrolytes.

The ATLS® recommends giving two litres of warmed physiological fluids (Hartmann's or Ringer's lactate) immediately, although some surgeons in the UK often start colloids (such as haemaccel) if there is definite blood loss. Obviously it is important to get the blood as soon as possible. O negative blood is used if necessary (the universal donor), whilst awaiting the X-match.

Recognize the signs of shock, and look for a cause. The chest, abdomen and pelvis are the likely causes if there is no obvious haemorrhage from a wound. A bleed into the abdomen causes distention and signs on examination, such as tenderness, guarding and maybe absent bowel sounds. If intraperitoneal bleeding is suspected (say, in a stab wound) and the patient is shocked despite immediate resuscitation, then no time should be wasted and the patient should be taken straight to theatre for a laparotomy to "turn off the tap". If the findings on examination are equivocal and the patient is not unstable, then a diagnostic peritoneal lavage (DPL), ultrasound or CT scan can be performed (in the USA an ultrasound is often available in casualty).

Diagnostic Peritoneal Lavage (DPL)

For finals you probably just need to know that this involves an incision in the mid-line, below the umbilicus, and dissection down to the peritoneum, into which a catheter is placed. A litre of normal saline is run into the peritoneal cavity. The bag is then placed on the floor and allowed to fill. If there is no obvious blood, then a sample of fluid is sent for microscopy to count the red blood cells. A urinary catheter and nasogastric tube must be inserted prior to the DPL in order to avoid damage to the stomach and bladder during the procedure. The findings of this procedure, however, are often very equivocal.

An unstable fractured pelvis can cause profuse blood loss and stage IV shock. The cause is usually venous bleeding. During the primary survey the chest and abdomen will have been examined to look for other causes of the shock. An orthopaedic surgeon can place an external fixator onto the pelvis, and this usually stops the rapid blood loss (by tamponade; and also stops any shearing forces on the vessels).

Disability

See section on head injury.

Exposure/Environment

The patient is completely exposed so that a full examination can be performed. In order to protect him from heat loss, he and the resus room should be heated. Methods for heating the patient include the use of warmed fluids and blood, and covering him with blankets. A *log roll* may be performed here, or it may be performed in the secondary survey. In this procedure one person holds and turns the head and neck and three people roll the body. This allows the patient to be turned with in-line cervical spine immobilization to examine the back of the body for any signs of trauma (stab wounds, bruising, abrasions), palpating for any tenderness, and a rectal examination is performed.

Secondary Survey

A quick history should be ascertained, from witnesses, family or the ambulancemen. The mnemonic AMPLE is used for the following vital questions:

Allergies
Medication

Past medical history
Last ate or drank
Events prior to the accident

The secondary survey is the head-to-toe or full examination. Check the head (eyes, ears, scalp — run your fingers through the hair), cervical spine, chest, abdomen, limbs, and make a full neurological examination. If the log roll has not been performed in the primary survey, it should be performed here.

At the end of the secondary survey the patient should be re-evaluated by starting again at the ABC's. Once you are sure he is fully stabilized you can begin to make arrangements for definitive care (this usually means an admission).

Cervical Spine — X-Rays and Management

A cervical spine injury is almost always accompanied by pain in the neck; however, it is important to know that the absence of a neurological deficit does not rule out a fracture of the cervical spine. Under A for "airway" with cervical spine control, the neck should be immobilized and a lateral "shoot through" X-ray should be taken. If a motorcycle helmet needs to be removed or intubation is required, these should be performed with in-line manual immobilization.

Assessment of the Cervical Spine X-Ray

Yet again think of the ABC's — Adequacy and alignment, Bones, Cartilages and Soft tissues. To get an acceptable film you should see the junction between the body of C7 and T1. If given a cervical spine X-ray in an exam and all you can see is C1-6, tell the examiner that this is not acceptable and you would like a further view. If he tells you that this is the best they could get and asks you what other methods you could use to improve the view, then say that you would like to repeat the X-ray with someone pulling down on the arms from the end of the bed or would like a swimmer's view (where the arm is abducted fully).

Alignment. Assess four lines — the line that runs down the anterior vertebral bodies, the anterior vertebral canal, the posterior vertebral canal and the tips of the spinous processes. These should be curved with a slight lordosis. A step along this line or a loss of the lordosis is abnormal. If the anteroposterior spinal canal space is narrowed, there is likely spinal cord compression.

Bone. Look at the shape of the individual vertebral bodies (which should be rectangular in shape), the lateral mass (the pedicles, facets, laminae and transvere processes) and the spinous processes.

Cartilage. Assess the intervertebral discs (should be of equal height) and facet joints.

Soft tissues. Just anterior to the vertebral bodies are the soft tissues of the pharynx. If there is damage to the cervical spine, there is likely to be associated soft tissue swelling (haemorrhage). Look at the shadow of the prevertebral space for any swelling. In front of the upper cervical vertebrae its normal width is about half that of the vertebral body (or less than 5 mm). At about C4 the soft tissues take up more space with a width about equal to that of the vertebral body (as the larynx and oesophagus are here). If the space between the spinous processes is widened, this implies a torn interspinous ligament.

SHOCK

Shock is defined as an inadequate perfusion and tissue oxygenation of the vital organs (brain, heart, kidneys and skin). There are several causes of shock and they can be divided into haemorrhagic and nonhaemorrhagic. The nonhaemorrhagic causes include cardiogenic, anaphylactic and septic shock (they should be known about but are not covered here). Tension pneumothorax can cause shock due to a mediastinal shift and impairment of the venous return.

Haemorrhagic Shock

Haemorrhage is the commonest cause of shock after injury. The most important step is to recognize and treat shock early even if the blood pressure is normal. As a rule any patient who is cool and tachycardic should be assumed to be shocked until proven otherwise. The normal adult blood volume is 7% of body weight (about 5 l for a 70 kg man), whereas in a child it is about 9% of body weight, or 80 ml per kg. The body has excellent compensatory mechanisms to deal with volume loss (although as age increases these mechanisms become less efficient), and there may be no changes in the blood pressure until the loss is considerable.

On examination you should assess the appearance of the patient, the pulse, blood pressure, pulse pressure (the difference between the systolic and the diastolic blood pressure), respiratory rate, capillary refill time (normally less than 2 s), mental status and urine output.

There are four stages of shock based on the percentage of blood loss. If you play tennis you will have no problem in recalling the percentages, as in they are the same as the tennis scoring system.

Stage I Shock (0–15%)

This is up to 750 ml blood loss (based on a 70 kg man). This is the group that catches people out, as signs of shock are minimal. The patient is usually a little anxious; however, the pulse rate is usually less than 100 and the blood pressure and pulse pressure are normal.

Stage II Shock (15–30%)

This is 750–1500 ml volume loss. Again the patient is anxious and the pulse is now above 100, with an increased respiratory rate. The systolic blood pressure is still usually maintained (by vasoconstriction and increased cardiac output); however, the pulse pressure is now decreased, mainly because of a rise in the diastolic pressure.

Stage III Shock (30–40%)

Up to 2000 ml. Now you see all the classic signs of inadequate perfusion, including a marked tachycardia and tachypnoea and a drop in the systolic blood pressure. There may be evidence of CNS impairment, such as confusion. It is therefore important to recognize shock in stages I and II in order to prevent the patient from going into stage III shock.

Stage IV Shock (Greater than 40%)

With a loss of greater than 2 l the condition is immediately life-threatening. The pulse is weak and thready, there is a significant drop in the systolic blood pressure (the diastolic blood pressure may be unrecordable), and the patient is pale, cold and clammy, with a depressed consciousness level.

	Stage I	*Stage II*	*Stage III*	*Stage IV*
Blood Loss (%)	< 15%	15–30%	30–40%	> 40%
Blood Loss (ml)	< 750	750–1500	1500–2000	> 2000
Consciousness	Slightly anxious	Agitated	Confused	Depressed
Pulse Rate	< 100	> 100	> 120	> 140
Blood Pressure	Normal	Normal	Decreased	Decreased
Pulse Pressure	Normal	Decreased	Decreased	Decreased
Respiratory Rate	14–20	20–30	30–40	> 35
Urine Output (ml/h)	> 30	20–30	< 20	None
Replacement	Crystalloid	Colloid	Colloid+Blood	Colloid+Blood

Under C for "circulation", two large bore cannulae (brown or grey) should be inserted, preferably one into each antecubital fossa. According to Poiseuille's law, flow is proportional to the fourth power of the internal radius of the tube and inversely proportional to the length, and so a short fat tube is essential (a central line, although important for monitoring, is usually long and very thin and hence not effective for fluid resuscitation). If IV access is difficult in the antecubital fossae, then a cutdown on the saphenous vein can be attempted (this is 2 cm above and anterior to the medial malleolus). In a child less than six years old, an interosseous needle can be used (this is a needle inserted directly into the bone, allowing access to the vascular marrow just below the knee, and can be used to replace blood and fluids in the same way as a venous cannula inserted into any other site).

Blood should be taken for laboratory analysis, including a cross-match, FBC, U & E's, glucose, toxicology studies and a pregnancy test in females of childbearing age. Blood gases are often useful at this stage. A central line (a catheter in a large central vein) may be inserted to help monitor fluid replacement or if cardiogenic shock is suspected.

Insertion of a Central Line

There are in use two approaches, into the subclavian (infraclavicular) or the internal jugular vein. A guide wire based on the Seldinger technique is employed. In the subclavian approach the patient is supine with the head down about 15° (this helps distend the neck veins and prevents an air embolism). The head should be supported by another helper if a cervical spine injury is suspected. An aseptic technique is used. Some local anaesthetic is infiltrated into the skin. A needle attached to a saline-filled syringe is introduced 1cm below the junction of the middle and inner thirds of the clavicle. The needle is advanced medially and slightly upwards behind the clavicle (aiming for the sternal notch) as the plunger is slowly withdrawn. When venous blood enters the syringe, the syringe is removed leaving the needle in the vein. A guide wire is inserted through the needle into the vein. The needle is removed, leaving the guide wire in the vein. The central line is then inserted over the guide wire and into the vein. The central line is fixed to the skin with a suture and is dressed. The central line can be connected to a manometer to measure the central venous pressure.

The internal jugular approach is similar. The carotid pulse is felt just anterior to the midpoint of the sternocleidomastoid muscle (the high approach) and a needle is inserted lateral to this, aiming posteroinferiorly and towards the nipple on that side (the internal jugular vein lies posterior to the carotid artery at the base of the skull; the vein then twists around the carotid and lies lateral to it half-way down the neck and in front of it just below the clavicle). In the low approach the needle is inserted between the two heads of sternocleidomastoid just above the clavicle.

After the central line is inserted it is important to get a check X-ray to identify the position of the line and a possible pneumothorax.

Complications of central line insertion include pneumothorax and haemopneumothorax (especially with the subclavian approach), arterial puncture (it is easier to apply pressure to the internal jugular artery if it is hit by mistake, whereas the subclavian is quite well hidden), haematoma formation and infection.

The ATLS® recommends starting two litres of crystalloid fluids as the initial resuscitation for every major trauma patient. The response to volume expansion is monitored by the same signs and symptoms that are used to diagnose it. The urine output is the best indicator of the adequacy of resuscitation.

There are three types of response to the initial fluid resuscitation:

(I)   *Rapid response*. Here the patients respond rapidly to the fluids and remain haemodynamically stable once the fluids are stopped or slowed. These patients have usually lost minimal blood volume (< 20%) and can be observed but do not necessarily need any further intravenous fluids.

(II) *Transient response*. There is an initial response with a rise in the blood pressure and a fall in the pulse rate; however, as the fluids are slowed down, the indices used to measure shock start to deteriorate again, indicating that the blood loss is ongoing or resuscitation has been inadequate. The response to the blood will indicate those patients who are still slowly bleeding (as may other clinical findings).

(III) *No response*. There is likely to be exsanguinating haemorrhage. Blood is needed rapidly. Type-specific blood (the ABO and Rhesus groups are compatible, but there may be some minor antibodies that are incompatible) takes about 10 min to process and should be given initially in life-threatening bleeding whilst waiting for the full cross-match, which takes maybe 40 min (as a last resort, Group O negative blood can be given). Failure to respond to the fluid resuscitation and the blood indicate the need for immediate surgical intervention to control the haemorrhage (turn off the tap). Very rarely, a failure of response may be due to the fact that there is a nonhaemorrhagic cause for the shock, such as myocardial contusion or tamponade, and a CVP measurement may help differentiate the causes.

If blood is given (usually packed red cells without plasma) it should be warmed to prevent hypothermia and, after a large transfusion, platelets and fresh frozen plasma may be needed to correct the lack of clotting factors. The main aim of transfusion is to correct the oxygen-carrying capacity, since crystalloids and colloids can both correct the lack of intravascular volume but have no oxygen-carrying capacity.

HEAD INJURIES

Introduction

Head injuries are common and range from the minor bump on the head that usually has the patient sent home with no investigation or treatment apart from advice, through to the multiply injured patient with an associated head injury and a depressed level of consciousness. The majority of head injuries fall somewhere between these two extremes, and the difficulty for the doctor is in deciding who needs to be admitted for observation and who can be sent home. Questions on head injuries are common in finals.

Anatomy

The scalp has five layers, described by the letters SCALP — Skin, Connective tissue, Aponeurosis, Loose connective tissue and Periosteum (pericraneum). It is highly vascular and can lead to large blood losses. Beneath the scalp is the skull, which contains the meninges, and then the brain. In a head injury any of these structures can be damaged.

The skull in an adult is a rigid structure that cannot expand. It contains cerebrospinal fluid (CSF), blood and the brain. If the volume of one of these components increases, then the other two must decrease to compensate or the intracranial pressure (the pressure that the CSF in the subarachnoid space is under) will rise.

This can be expressed by a formula based on the modified Monroe–Kellie hypothesis:

$$K_{ICP} \sim V_{CSF} + V_{Bl} + V_{Br}.$$

Constancy (K) of the intracranial pressure (ICP) relates to the volume (V) of the CSF plus the volume of the blood (Bl) plus the volume of the brain (Br). The ICP is usually maintained at a constant level by excellent autoregulatory mechanisms that can accommodate changes in the blood flow. For example, the CSF has a particular relationship with CO_2 , in that rises in CO_2 cause an increase in the cerebral blood flow.

Large increases in the ICP lead to a decrease in the cerebral perfusion pressure (CPP), which is a measure of the amount of oxygenated blood reaching the brain:

$$CPP = Mean\ systemic\ BP - ICP.$$

(Normally this is greater than 40 mmHg, and if less than that you get first electrical and then structural brain damage). In the presence of an expanding haematoma within the skull, the autoregulatory mechanisms can initially accommodate this. The first response is for venous blood and the CSF (or both) to be displaced out of the cranial cavity. We can accommodate a mass of about 50–100 ml

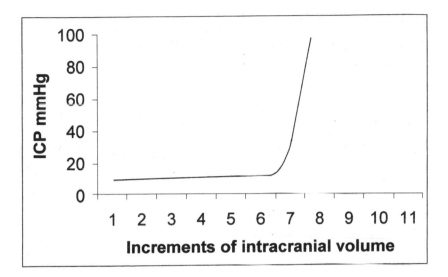

Figure 4.1. Graph of intracranial volume against intracranial pressure. Note that the pressure rises very rapidly after a period of compensation when fluid is squeezed out of the CSF spaces and venous sinuses.

without a significant rise in the ICP. However, as the mass expands further, the autoregulatory mechanisms fail and the rise in the ICP is rapid (as is the patient's deterioration) and can lead to brain herniation.

Types of Injury

(I) **Scalp Laceration**
   Lacerations of the scalp can bleed profusely and lead to major blood loss, especially in children.

(II) **Skull Fracture**
   Skull fractures are common. It is possible to have one without severe brain injury, and likewise you can have an intracranial injury without accompanying skull fracture, especially in children, whose bones are more supple. The only significance of X-raying head injuries

and looking for a skull fracture is that such patients have a statistically higher probability of developing a bleed into the brain, and hence they get admitted for observation. The types of fracture are:

- *Linear (nondepressed) fracture.* This appears as a lucent line.
- *Depressed skull fracture.* Management will depend on the underlying brain injury. The fragment may need to be elevated if depressed more than the thickness of the skull or if there are focal signs.
- *Open skull fracture.* This usually requires operative intervention. A broad spectrum antibiotic should be started, the patient taken to theatre for wound debridement and the fracture dealt with.
- *Basal skull fracture.* This fracture cannot usually be seen on a plain X-ray of the skull, although it should be suspected if there are fluid levels in the sphenoidal sinuses. The diagnosis is made on clinical findings of the CSF leaking from the nose (rhinorrhoea) or the ears (otorrhoea). The CSF is usually crystal-clear, unless it is blood-stained. It can be tested for by allowing a drop to fall onto a piece of filter paper. The blood remains at the centre and the CSF soaks around it in concentric rings of clear fluid, called the "halo sign".

Other clinical signs of a basal skull fracture include the *battle sign* — bruising around the mastoid region due to tracking of blood under the skin, and haemotympanum (blood behind the tympanic membrane), which together with CSF otorrhoea are indicative of a middle fossa fracture through the petrous temporal bone. The *badger sign* (bruising around both orbits), together with rhinorrhoea, is associated with a fracture of the cribriform plate. The badger and battle signs may, however, take several hours to develop.

(III) **Brain Injury**
Injuries to the brain can be primary, occurring at the time of impact; or secondary, caused by hypovolaemia, hypoxia, hypo-glycaemia

and raised intracranial pressure. Prevention of primary brain injury can only be brought about by measures to stop the accident happening in the first place, such as having road speed limits and the wearing of motorcycle helmets. The main aim in the management of a head injury is, therefore, to prevent or limit the damage that occurs because of the secondary injury.

The types of primary brain damage can be diffuse or focal.

Diffuse Injuries

- *Concussion*. This is a brain injury accompanied by a temporary loss of neurological function. The changes are reversible and are often resolved by the time the patient arrives in hospital. He may have just been confused or dazed at the scene or may have lost consciousness. Afterwards he may complain of a headache, feel dizzy, be amnesic or nauseous, and generally if the patient has been unconscious for more than five minutes it is probably best to admit him to hospital for observation.
- *Diffuse axonal injury*. This is a more severe injury, with microscopic structural damage throughout the brain tissue. It is often characterized by prolonged coma and can last from days to weeks. Such patients can develop autonomic dysfunction and hence have high fevers, hypertension and sweating. The mortality is high.

Focal Injuries

- *Contusions*. These are focal areas of brain injury. They can be *coup* injuries, where the brain is damaged directly by the skull at the point of impact; or *contre coup* injuries, where the brain is squashed by the skull at a remote point from the impact.

  The patient may have a focal neurological deficit, depending on the site of the contusion. Oedema may develop at the site of damage and cause a neurological deterioration. The patient is usually managed conservatively; however, because of the risk of delayed bleeding into the contusion, he needs to be observed carefully for deterioration (especially in alcoholics).

- **Intracranial haemorrhage**. This can be meningeal or into the brain tissue.

Acute extradural/epidural haemorrhage. This is due to a bleed from the arteries that supply the skull and dura — usually the middle meningeal artery, which sits just under the skull in a region called the pterion (or temple). This type of bleed is quite rare, accounting for less than 1% of coma-producing head injuries; however, it can be rapidly fatal. There is usually an associated skull fracture of the parietal or temporal bone often caused by a direct blow — for example, being hit over the side of the head by a baseball bat.

The typical picture is:

Loss of consciousness (concussion), followed by a lucid interval. During this lucid interval the haematoma is expanding into the extradural space and compressing the brain inwards, stripping the dura off the skull as it expands (hence the convex appearance of the clot on the CT). As mentioned before, the ICP does not rise initially as the mass is accommodated; however, once the clot reaches a critical volume the ICP increases rapidly.

The rapid rise in the ICP causes a secondary lapse in the consciousness level.

As the ICP rises further the uncus (the medial aspect of the temporal lobe) herniates through the tentorium (the layer that divides the cerebral hemispheres from the brain stem and cerebellum). The third nerve passes through this opening and can be compressed at this point. The patient initially develops a constriction of the pupil on the affected side, which then begins to dilate up (Hutchinson's pupil). The fixed dilated pupil on the affected side is usually accompanied by a hemiparesis on the opposite side (the corticospinal fibres cross over). As the pressure continues to increase, the opposite pupil dilates up and eventually the brain stem "cones" through the foramen magnum.

This injury requires immediate surgical intervention. The patient should have a CT as early as possible if this type of injury is suspected. Neurosurgical advice should be sought and the patient transferred if necessary for surgical evacuation of the clot. If the injury is treated early the prognosis is excellent.

Acute subdural haemorrhage. This is much more common than an extradural haemorrhage, and occurs in about 30% of severe head injuries. It is usually due to rupture of a bridging vein between the cerebral cortex and the dura (but it can also be due to laceration of the cerebral cortex), and is often caused by a rotational injury. The elderly are more susceptible, as their brains are often shrunken and hence the bridging veins are put under tension. The bleeding is typically less brisk than an extradural haemorrhage, but clinically it can present with symptoms of an expanding mass as above. The prognosis is much worse and the mortality high.

Subarachnoid haemorrhage. This can be associated with trauma, although it is usually due to hypertension and bleeding from berry aneurysms. The symptoms are those of meningeal irritation similar to meningitis.

Brain haemorrhages and lacerations. These are tears to the brain substance with bleeding into them. The deficit will depend on the site of the damage. These injuries are therefore similar to strokes, and surgery cannot help the patient. Rehabilitation can be very slow.

Assessment of Severe Head Injuries

As the patient is brought into casualty you should attempt to get some history, finding out as much as possible about the incident. If he is unconscious the history is taken from witnesses or the ambulance crew, etc. Falls from a height should be taken very seriously, as they have a much greater risk of an intracranial bleed than road traffic accidents. For a fall, inquire about the height of the fall and whether it was onto concrete or grass, etc. If the patient was driving a car, inquire about the speed of the car and whether a seat-belt was worn, whether any of the other passengers were injured or dead, and whether alcohol or drugs were involved. Was consciousness lost? If so, for how long? Has the patient regained consciousness since the accident or has he remained unconscious ever since? Has the patient fitted since or complained of visual disturbances, dizziness or a worsening headache?

Perform the primary survey according to ATLS® guidelines — ABCDE.

The *Glasgow Coma Score* (GCS) is a quantitative measure the patient's level of consciousness. It is divided into three parts: assessing the best motor response, the best eye opening response and the best verbal response. It was devised to allow comparisons to be made (if necessary by different observers) to see if the patient's consciousness has improved or deteriorated. The minimum score is 3 and the maximum 15.

A Glasgow Coma Score (GCS) of 8 or less implies coma and a severe head injury. If the score is greater than 8, then the patient is not in a coma. A GCS of between 9 and 12 implies a moderate head injury and a GCS of 13–15 shows a minor head injury.

The GCS should be repeated at regular intervals, and a deterioration by more than two points should be taken very seriously and a neurosurgical consultation sought.

Assess the vital signs. Remember that although bleeding from a scalp wound can cause shock, bleeding into the skull cannot, and therefore never assume that hypotension is due to an intracranial bleed, or to brain injury (as this is a terminal event on failure of the medullary centres). Look for another cause.

The Cushing response is a combination of progressive hypertension, bradycardia and a decreased respiratory rate (the opposite of hypovolaemic shock). It is due to a lethal rise in the ICP, usually by an intracranial bleed needing urgent decompression.

Table of GCS (Glasgow Coma Score)

Best Eye Opening	Score
Spontaneous	4
To voice	3
To pain	2
None	1

Best Verbal Response	Score
Orientated	5
Confused	4
Inappropriate speech	3
Incomprehensible speech	2
No speech	1

Best Motor Response	Score
Obeys commands	6
Localizes to pain	5
Withdraws from pain	4
Flexes to pain	3
Extension to pain	2
None	1
Total	3–15

Hypertension alone or with hyperthermia suggests central autonomic dysfunction caused by diffuse brain injury.

Under D for "disability", document the patient's AVPU score. If the airway, breathing and circulation are under control, then the minineurological examination can be performed in the primary survey; otherwise it is performed in the secondary survey.

The minineurological examination involves three components:

(1) Level of consciousness — the Glasgow Coma Score.

(2) Pupillary function — are the pupils equal and reactive to light?
(3) Lateralizing neurology — swiftly assess the tone, power and reflexes of all four limbs.

The purpose of this is to detect those with a severe head injury who are likely to need surgery (i.e. those with abnormalities of all three components).

Remember that the initial neurological examination is only a baseline for comparing the results of repeated examinations, in order to determine deterioration or improvement of the patient's condition.

Management of Severe Head Injuries

This involves, firstly, dealing with the life-threatening injuries (ABC); then, assessing the severity of the head injury, whilst preventing secondary brain damage from occurring, by ensuring optimal cerebral metabolic supplies and preventing intracranial hypertension.

Cerebral Metabolism

The brain requires oxygen and glucose to function, and so adequate substrates must be present in the circulation to supply this need. The oxygen content depends on both the arterial haemoglobin and the PO_2. The PO_2 can be measured by blood gases, and oxygen supplemented as necessary. If the haemoglobin is low a transfusion may be required to improve the oxygen-carrying capacity.

Raised Intracranial Pressure

This may be due to a mass lesion or brain oedema, and should be treated.

Cerebral blood flow is dependent on both the arterial PCO_2 and the systemic blood pressure. As the arterial PCO_2 rises cerebrovasodilatation occurs, worsening the raised ICP. In reverse, reducing the arterial PCO_2

reduces the cerebral blood volume and hence the intracranial pressure. Therefore, in cases of raised ICP the patient should be hyperventilated to keep the PCO_2 low. To do this it is usually necessary to intubate and ventilate the patient. So early involvement of an anaesthetist is essential, firstly to secure the airway and then to help hyperventilate. Remember that a decrease in the PCO_2 leads to a decrease in the cerebral blood flow and so the PCO_2 must be kept at about 3.5 as a compromise.

Intravenous fluids may be needed in the management of other problems, such as shock, and the risk is that overhydration may make cerebral oedema worse. Therefore isotonic fluids such as Hartmann's should be administered rather than hyposmolar fluids such as dextrose.

Diuretics such as mannitol are often used to reduce intracranial pressure, and are given if a mass lesion is suspected whilst awaiting transfer to a neurosurgical unit, although a neurosurgical consultation should be obtained prior to giving any diuretics (if diuretics are used a urinary catheter is required to aid fluid balance measurement). Steroids have no place in the acute management of head injury.

Management of Mild to Moderate Head Injuries

The problem for a casualty officer when he sees what appears to be a minor head injury is in deciding who needs admitting for observation. In general the history is important; one needs to know the mechanism of the injury. For example, was the patient the driver of the car, was he wearing a seat-belt, were any of the other passengers injured, was there a loss of consciousness and for how long, and was alcohol involved? Has the patient fitted since or complained of visual disturbances, dizziness or a worsening headache? Document the amnesia, for the events that led up to the incident (retrograde amnesia) or for the events that followed the incident (anterograde amnesia). The length of anterograde amnesia has been shown to be a good indicator of the severity of the head injury (less than 1 h — mild; 1–24 h — moderate; more than 24 h — severe), although this is not much help in the initial assessment, which takes place soon after the incident. With children it is also worth noting whether they cried immediately, as this is a good sign (normal behaviour), or whether they were limp and unresponsive.

Examination is essentially the same as above; however, in some cases it is difficult to decide what investigations are needed and whether or not you can safely send the patient home. For example, let us say the patient has walked into the department after a head injury sustained in an assault where he was hit over the head by a brick. His speech is slurred from drink and he has a bump on his forehead, but there is no focal neurology to find on examination (within the limits of the cooperation of this patient). A large proportion of patients present like this. Do you X-ray these patients?

X-rays may help in deciding who will be admitted for observation, but not much else. If there is a skull fracture, then the risk of an intracranial bleed is significantly higher.

Rough risk of intracranial haematoma in adults

	No Skull Fracture	*Skull Fracture*
Fully Conscious	< 1/1000	1/30
Depressed Consciousness	1/100	1/4

Therefore the indications for doing an X-ray are as follows:

(1) Loss of consciousness for more than a few minutes.
(2) Neurological symptoms or signs (unless a CT is indicated) such as visual disturbances, dizziness, weakness, persistent vomiting, etc.
(3) Signs of a basal skull fracture.
(4) Suspected penetrating injuries (X-rays are essential in this case).
(5) Common sense, i.e. history of significant injury or obvious significant scalp wound.
(6) When there is difficulty in assessing the patient (young/old, drunk, postepileptic).

In the example given above it may be sensible to X-ray the patient, as he is drunk and such patients are difficult to assess. If there is a skull fracture he will be admitted for observation. If there is no skull fracture you may allow him to go home, providing he is with someone sensible who can observe him.

The indications for admission are:

(1) Skull fracture.
(2) Depressed level of consciousness or confusion when examined.
(3) Neurological symptoms or signs.
(4) Difficult to assess.
(5) Social circumstances; patient lives alone, with no responsible adult to observe him.

If the patient is admitted, he is usually given nonopiate analgesia (or codeine phosphate, which is safe to use) and taken to the ward, and regular neurological observations are performed, at first hourly. The observations include the vital signs, the GCS, pupils and motor function, and are represented schematically on a graph to detect any deterioration.

If the patient is not admitted he should be sent home with head injury instructions (go to your casualty department and get a copy) to stay with a responsible adult who will bring him back should his condition deteriorate.

BURNS

Different types of burns tend to affect different age groups. Toddlers tend to be scalded, for example, by pulling the kettle wire or the pan off the stove, kids tend to set their clothes on fire, and the old tend to suffer domestic accidents at home. The majority of adult burns, however, are associated with industrial accidents (or are drug- or alcohol-related).

Pathology

The damage is caused by coagulation of proteins with cell death. The burn can affect any depth of skin. The superficial burn causes vasodilatation with diffuse erythema, kinins are released and pain is felt. As the depth increases, the capillaries become damaged and therefore more permeable, leading to blistering and oedema formation. As the dermis becomes involved, the nerve endings which lie here are damaged and sensation is lost. Once the germinal layer is damaged, the skin will never regrow, and these burns heal with fibrosis and contractures. The damaged necrotic tissue lying in a protein-rich exudate is an ideal medium for infection.

The increased capillary permeability can lead to the exudation of protein-rich fluid from the surface of the burn and oedema into the surrounding tissues. The patient can very quickly become hypovolaemic.

Types of Burns

(1) Thermal — can be dry (fire) or wet (scald)
(2) Chemical
(3) Electrical
(4) Friction

Chemical burns. These result from exposure to acids, alkalis or petroleum products. In general, alkali burns are more serious than acid burns as they penetrate more deeply. The chemical should be flushed away from the skin with copious amounts of irrigation with water (20–30 min). If dry powder is present brush it away before irrigating. The neutralizing agents are no better than water.

Electrical burns. These are more serious than they appear. The overlying skin may look normal, but deeper tissue may be damaged. Rhabdomyolysis leads to myoglobin release and the risk of acute renal failure. The patient can also develop cardiac disturbance due to acidosis and changes in potassium concentration. A cardiac monitor and a urinary catheter are therefore necessary. The patient will have dark urine due to the myoglobin and require large amounts of fluids to ensure a high urine output. If necessary, mannitol can be used to maintain a diuresis and flush out the myoglobin.

Management of the Burns Patient

The management of the burns patient, as with any trauma patient, is to exclude any life-threatening injuries first (i.e. ABCDE, according to ATLS® guidelines).

The main priorities with burns patients, however, are:

(1) Securing the airway
(2) Management of fluid loss
(3) Prevention of infection

Immediate Resuscitation

Secure the airway, and stop the burning process by removing all clothing.

Airway

The supraglottic airway can rapidly become obstructed due to oedema and swelling following a burn injury. It is therefore important to suspect involvement of the airway, even if the patient is breathing normally when first examined. Apart from the obvious signs of airway injury, such as stridor or hoarseness, any of the following should alert the doctor to the likely presence of an acute inhalation injury:

(1) Facial burns
(2) Singeing of the eyebrows or nasal hairs
(3) Carbonaceous sputum
(4) Altered consciousness
(5) History — such as long exposure to smoke or gases, or an explosion.

An anaesthetist must be called immediately. Early endotracheal intubation is better than adopting a wait-and-see policy, as the airway can be obstructed rapidly.

Breathing

Apart from direct thermal injury, which causes upper airway oedema and obstruction, inhalation of toxic fumes and smoke can lead to chemical tracheobronchitis, oedema and pneumonia. You should always assume carbon monoxide (CO) exposure if the patient is confined to an enclosed area.

CO has an affinity for haemoglobin that is about 240 times that of oxygen, and hence oxygen is displaced and the oxygen dissociation curve is shifted to the left. The CO dissociates very slowly when the patient is breathing room air, with a half-life of about 6 h. If 100% oxygen is breathed the half-life is shortened to about 40 min. Therefore, the patient should have arterial blood gases taken for assessment of the carboxyhaemoglobin concentration and 100% oxygen should be commenced. He may have a headache, nausea, vomiting, or confusion at high levels of exposure, but the classic cherry-red skin appearance is rare.

Circulation

It may be difficult to get a reliable blood pressure owing to the burns, and the urine output is probably the best indicator of circulating blood volume.

Establish intravenous access if necessary through the burnt skin, and start two litres of Hartmann's solution immediately. The fluid losses can be huge and a 50% burns patient can lose up to half his plasma volume in about 3–4 h.

A rough guide is to replace 2–4 ml of crystalloid fluid for each kilogram body weight per percentage burn in the first 24 h. So a 70 kg man with a 50% burn will require between 7 and 14 l in the first 24 h ($2 \times 70 \times 50 = 7000$ ml $= 7$ l). Half the fluid should be given in the first 8 h from the time of the burn (not the time of arrival to casualty), so if the burn was 2 h before arrival, he will need at a very minimum 3.5 l in the next 6 h.

In some departments the policy is to replace colloids such as human albumin solution (HAS), and in this case the Muir and Barclay formula can be used. This determines how much plasma volume is needed in terms of colloid replacement.

Volume of colloid needed (per unit time)
$$= \text{Weight (kg)} \times \text{percentage burn}/2 \, .$$

So, for a 70 kg man, with a 50% burn this would be 1.75 l of colloid per unit time ($70 \times 50/2 = 1750$ ml). The first amount in the first 4 h from the burn, then the same amount in the subsequent 4 h, 4 h, 6 h, 6 h and 12 h. This would total about 8.75 l of colloid in the first day and in addition crystalloid maintenance (about 3 l) with, say, normal saline is required.

Remember that these figures are just guides and whether crystalloids or colloids have been given the best indicator of sufficient replacement is an adequate urine output of greater than 30–50 ml per hour. The haematocrit is also used to guide fluid balance.

Circumferential full thickness burns to the limbs can impede the blood supply owing to oedema in a confined space (a tourniquet effect), and are best treated by escharotomies (an incision through scar tissue). The incision is made along the line of the limb through the entire scar. As this is a full thickness burn, sensation is absent and in theory no anaesthetic is required. In practice, however, the escharotomy tends to be done with the patient anaesthetized (there are some areas of partial thickness burns adjacent to the full thickness zones and the escharotomy can therefore be painful when these areas are cut). Cross-matched blood must be available, as this procedure can bleed profusely.

Circumferential burns of the thorax may cause restriction of chest expansion, and bilateral escharotomies may be needed.

Assessing the Burn (History, Size and Depth of the Burn)

History

Note the cause and exact time of the burn (remember to ask about associated injuries — for example, did the patient jump out of a window to escape the fire?). Try to ascertain some past medical history, such as diabetes, hypertension, heart or lung disease, the medication the patient is on, allergies and tetanus status.

Depth of Burn

Superficial burns (also called first degree burns) are not life-threatening and are simply painful red areas, such as sunburn. There is no blistering.

Partial thickness burns (also called second degree burns) — here there is associated swelling and blistering, and the skin is red and may be oozing fluid. These burns are very painful even to air current.

Full thickness burns (also called third degree burns) — the skin is dry, painless and insensate; it may appear pale, white or charred.

Body Surface Area (BSA)

The "rule of nines" is a useful way to determine the extent of the burn. The adult body is divided into regions that represent 9% of the body area.

The genital region is considered to be 1% of the BSA.

The proportions are different in children whose head contributes more than the legs to the total area (as it does for heat loss).

Another good guide is that the *patient's* palm (not your palm and not including the patient's fingers) represents about 1% of the body surface area.

You can use these guides to estimate that, in an adult with a burn to one arm and one leg with a small area affected on the torso of about three palm sizes, the percentage burn will be about 30% (9 + 18 + 3).

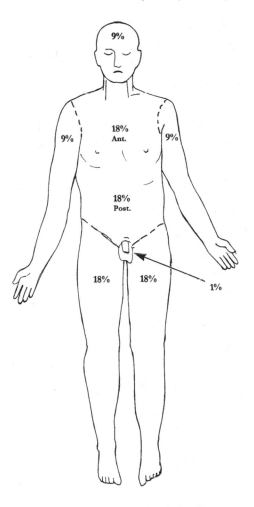

Figure 4.2. The "rule of nines".

Summary of Management of the Burns Patient

(1) Airway — look for signs of obstruction or signs indicating the risk of obstruction; inform the anaesthetist.
(2) Breathing — pulse oximetry; look for signs of CO poisoning, 100% oxygen, arterial blood gas analysis; request a chest X-ray.
(3) Circulation — IV access × 2

      — take blood for FBC, U&E's, glucose, X-match, carboxyhaemoglobin levels.

      — Start IV fluids, ECG; catheterize if necessary.

(4) Assess the burn depth and body surface area, adjust fluid requirements, consider escharotomies.

(5) Analgesia — opiates titrated to the patient's pain.

(6) Assess for associated injuries; a nasogastric tube may be needed.

(7) Cover the burns — partial thickness burns are painful to air current; gently cover them with sterile towels. Do not apply any antiseptic and do not pierce the blisters.

(8) Take extra special precautions to avoid infection, which after the initial resuscitation is the main cause of morbidity and mortality.

The patient should be transferred to a regional burns unit if necessary, especially if:

(I)   There is a partial thickness burn of greater than 15% BSA (in the very young or old a 10% burn should be referred).

(II)   Full thickness burn of greater than 5%.

(III) Involvement of the face, hands, feet, genitalia or over major joints.

(IV) Significant chemical or electrical burns.

The burns should be covered with clingfilm, then put warm blankets over them before transfer as the use of agents such as sulphasalizine or paraffin gauze interfere with the assessment of the burn when the patient arrives at the burns unit.

5

LIVER, BILIARY TREE AND PANCREAS

Many of the pathological entities in this section appear in both medicine and surgery, and questions on them may therefore be found in either part of the finals examination. There is, however, often a different emphasis between the type of answer one should give in a medical examination and in a surgical examination, even when dealing with the same condition. Having said that, however, most surgeons now work closely with their physician colleagues and, despite differences of emphasis, will usually have similar views about management and the precise role of surgical intervention.

INVESTIGATIONS

The relevant investigations for most conditions of the liver, biliary tree and pancreas are blood tests (including liver function tests), ultrasound and CT or MRI scans, which are used to give more details of liver lesions or to look at the lower end of the bile duct and pancreas, where ultrasound often gives poor views because of overlying bowel gas. An additional test is the ERCP (Endoscopic Retrograde CholangioPancreatogram), which is done by using a special endoscope passed through the mouth into the second part of the duodenum. The ampulla of Vater (the place where the pancreatic and the common bile duct open into the duodenum) can be identified and cannulated, and X-rays of the pancreatic duct and biliary tree are taken after injection of contrast media. As well as being an investigation, the ERCP offers the possibility of therapeutic manoeuvres such as sphincterotomy (i.e. cutting the sphincter to widen it), stone extraction or stent insertion.

Liver Function Tests

These usually consist of:

Bilirubin	A rise of bilirubin is the definition of "jaundice". It is bilirubin which makes the patient yellow.
Alkaline phosphastase	This enzyme tends to be raised more with obstruction of the bile ducts (i.e. "obstructive jaundice").
Transaminases (e.g. ALT, AST)	These tend to be raised more with defective liver cell function (i.e. "hepatocellular function").
Albumin	This synthesised by the liver and is low in chronic liver disease and malnutrition.
Gamma GT	This enzyme is raised in both hepatocellular and obstructive liver disorders.

In addition, the prothrombin time or INR (INR = international ratio, i.e. the length of time the patient's blood takes to clot in comparison with a normal person's) may be abnormal and should be checked in any jaundiced patient or when defective liver synthesis is suspected. If abnormal it can be corrected by vitamin K (vitamin K is a fat-soluble vitamin and is not absorbed well in many forms of liver disease because of a lack of bile salts, which are required to emulsify fats in the intestinal lumen).

GALLSTONES

Gallstones are very common and are therefore frequently asked about in finals. The majority are asymptomatic and require no treatment. They can, however, cause a wide range of clinical problems, depending on their position (see table). They are either made up of cholesterol and pigment (composed of bilirubin breakdown products) or a mixture of the two. Pure pigment stones are rare (< 10%) and are found in conditions such as haemolytic anaemia. Most (75%) gallstones are predominantly cholesterol. Ninety per cent of gallstones are radio-lucent, i.e. they do not show on a plain X-ray (unlike renal calculi, of which 90% are radio-opaque). Predisposing factors to gallstone formaton include female sex (three times more common), obesity , age (10% of >50-year-olds have gallstones, and 30% of >70-year-olds), haemolytic anemia, hyperlipidaemias and Crohn's disease. Some people also appear to have an innate tendency to form gallstones and are said to have "lithogenic bile". People often refer to the typical gallstone patient as fat, female, fertile and forty.

Complications of gallstones

(A) *In the Gallbladder*
  (i)   Chronic cholecystitis
  (ii) Biliary colic
  (iii) Acute cholecystitis
    • Empyaema
    • Biliary peritonitis
    • Abscess
  (iv) Mucocele
  (v) Carcinoma of gallbladder

(B) *In the Common Bile Duct*
  (i)   Obstructive jaundice
  (ii) Cholangitis
  (iii) Pancreatitis

(C) *In the Gut*
  (i)   Gallstone ileus

CHRONIC CHOLECYSTITIS

Chronic cholecystitis is a term used to describe symptoms of upper abdominal pain, indigestion, bloating, burping, nausea and occasional vomiting. Sometimes this symptom complex is called flatulent dyspepsia. The patient may describe the symptoms as being precipitated by fatty food (fats stimulate the release of cholecystokinin, which causes gallbladder contractions). There is usually nothing to find on physical examination. The main differential diagnoses include peptic ulceration, hiatus hernia and irritable bowel syndrome. Because gallstones are common it is important not to automatically ascribe such symptoms to them simply because gallstones are present on an ultrasound scan. A missed peptic ulcer or irritable bowel syndrome will obviously not be helped by unnecessary cholecystectomy and the patient will continue to get symptoms (sometimes called postcholecystectomy syndrome). If the symptoms are thought to be arising from the gallbladder and are significant, then the treatment is cholecystectomy, either open or laparoscopic. Attempts to dissolve gallstones using bile salt therapy are possible only in patients with small, noncalcified stones and are reserved for those who refuse or are unfit for surgery.

BILIARY COLIC

Biliary colic is the pain caused by gallbladder muscle spasms against a stone stuck in the neck of the gallbladder (Hartmann's pouch) or the cystic duct. It may account for some of the symptoms of chronic cholecystitis. Unlike intestinal colic, the pain is continuous and not in waves. It is usually felt in the epigastrium or right upper quadrant and may radiate around both costal margins and into the back. The pain can be extremely severe and patients may be sweaty, pale and tachycardic because of it. They may also feel nauseated or vomit. They will usually be unable to get comfortable and will prefer to writhe around rather than stay still. Attacks usually last less than 6 h and examination is usually otherwise normal. Differential diagnoses include other causes of severe upper abdominal pain, such as perforated peptic ulcer, pancreatitis, ruptured aneurysm, etc. Management involves giving analgesia, investigation to confirm gallstones (ultrasound) and subsequent cholecystectomy in most cases.

ACUTE CHOLECYSTITIS

In its earliest stage this may appear to be biliary colic, and indeed many attacks of acute cholecystitis probably start with biliary colic. Most episodes of acute cholecystitis are caused by chemical inflammation within an obstructed gallbladder and the exact mechanisms are poorly understood. Bacterial infection probably is a secondary event in about 1/3 of cases and these may be the ones most likely to develop complications. Patients will typically have severe right upper quadrant or epigastric pain. Like biliary colic, this may radiate around the costal margins or into the back. Unlike biliary colic, patients will prefer to lie still and take shallow breaths (this is now a form of local peritonitis, not a colic). They will usually have a temperature and tachycardia, and may also have nasuea and vomiting. Murphy's sign may be positive and is often asked about in vivas. It is elicited by pressing in the right upper quadrant under the costal margin. The patient is then asked to breathe in, and winces or gasps with pain as the gallbladder moves down and hits the examiner's hand. The test should also be performed in the left upper quadrant to exclude nonspecific reactions due to other pathology.

A mass may be present in the right upper quadrant, but if so this is not usually the gallbladder itself but rather a "phlegmon" (i.e. inflamed and adherent omentum and bowel around the gallbladder).

The treatment of acute cholecystitis is initial resuscitation with intravenous fluids and antibiotics. The patient will normally be kept nil by mouth or on sips of clear fluids, and initial investigations will be arranged, including basic blood tests such as an FBC (usually the white cell count is raised), U&E's, LFT's and amylase (as pancreatitis may be a differential diagnosis). The most important confirmatory test is usually an ultrasound scan. This can confirm gallstones, show thickening and oedema of the gallbladder wall and localise the tender spot to the gallbladder itself. It can also exclude dilatation of the common bile duct and other pathology, such as liver masses. Only very occasionally is a HIDA scan used to help confirm or exclude cholecystitis. The principle of this test is that HIDA (a radioisotope) is taken up by the liver and excreted into the bile. If the cystic duct is patent it will fill the gallbladder effectively, excluding cholecystitis.

With conservative treatment approximately 80–90% of cases of acute cholecystitis will settle over the next 24–48 h (i.e. the pain settles, the temperature falls and the patient's abdomen becomes nontender). In about 10% there will not be a prompt resolution of symptoms and signs, and in these cases surgery is usually advised. Particularly worrying signs are increasing temperature, tachycardia and the onset of increasing tenderness or the signs of peritonitis. These may indicate infarction of the gallbladder ("gangrenous cholecystitis") or perforation, which may produce either a local collection or generalised peritonitis. A gallbladder full of pus (empyaema of the gallbladder) usually leads to an unwell patient with the signs of sepsis (fever, tachycardia, hypotension, etc.) as well as pain, and tenderness in the right upper quadrant.

More controversial is the question of what to do with cases who do not absolutely require early surgery. Some surgeons prefer to perform a cholecystectomy during the episode of acute cholecystitis to remove the source of the problem. The conventional wisdom is that it should be done within three days of the onset of symptoms, because after this time the surgery becomes much more difficult because of adhesions and oedema and friability of tissues. An additional factor to consider is that most surgeons now prefer to perform laparoscopic cholecystectomy rather than open cholecytectomy, and this is definitiely more difficult in acute cholecystitis and indeed many surgeons consider acute cholecytitis to be a contraindication to laparoscopic cholecystectomy. Because of these considerations many units discharge their patients to be readmitted for an elective cholecystectomy 6–8 weeks later, at a time when the inflammation should have settled.

CHOLECYSTECTOMY

Laparoscopic cholecystectomy has now replaced open cholecystectomy in the majority of cases. Open cholecystectomy may still be indicated in difficult cases or when laparoscopic cholecystectomy has been attempted and has failed. It is usually performed through an upper midline or right subcostal incision. The cystic duct and the cystic artery are identified, ligated and divided (there is no cystic vein). The gallbladder is dissected free from the liver. Great care must be taken not to damage the bile duct.

The first laparoscopic cholecystectomy was performed in 1987 by Phillipe Mouret (a gynaecologist!) in France and the procedure has since become accepted as the mainstay treatment of uncomplicated gallstone disease. The term "laparoscopy" (peritoneoscopy) means a rigid endoscope is introduced into the peritoneal cavity, which is insufflated with a gas to lift off the anterior abdominal wall. The laparoscopic cholecystectomy is the best example of minimal access surgery (MAS) at the present time. MAS is essentially the same operation through a smaller wound. It encompasses laparoscopy, thoracoscopy, arthroscopy and endoluminal endoscopy. Although these techniques have been around for many years it is only within the last decade that laparoscopy has been used for surgical procedures such as laparoscopic cholecystectomy, colectomy, appendicectomy, hernia repair, etc.

Many would regard the other procedures as controversial and it would seem that with improved technology, expertise and training, many of these procedures will in the future become as widely accepted as laparoscopic cholecystectomy.

The proposed advantages of laparoscopic surgery are attributable to a smaller wound, and there will thus be less postoperative pain, the wound will heal quicker with less chance of infection, the patient will recover and mobilize quicker, return home sooner and hence return to work quicker.

The disadvantages of laparoscopy include the need for special equipment and extra training, the procedure itself is technically more challenging (hand–eye coordination), the complications are harder to deal with (e.g. haemostasis — the blood obscures the field of vision), and there is loss of tactile feedback. Recently there have been reports of tumour implantation at port hole sites, leaving questions unanswered as to the role of laparoscopic techniques in the management of malignant disease. The question as to whether laparoscopic surgery is cheaper and quicker or slower and more expensive involves so many factors (the expertise of the surgeon, the length of the operations, the cost of the shorter hospital stay, etc.) that it is probably best just to say that this remains controversial.

There are relatively few contraindications to laparoscopy, although patients with cardiac or respiratory problems do not tolerate the pneumoperitoneum well owing to a decreasd venous return and increased strain on the heart. Patients with bleeding disorders are best avoided, as bleeding is more difficult to deal with, and also patients who are shocked must have an open operation. Relative contraindications include those patients with multiple previous abdominal scars who are likely to have multiple adhesions between the bowel and the anterior abdominal wall, making laparoscopy hazardous. Pregnancy, certainly in the later stages, is also a relative contraindication.

The principles of laparoscopic cholecystectomy are as follows. A Verres needle is inserted into the peritoneal cavity, usually at the umbilicus. A pneumoperitoneum is created as the peritoneal cavity is insufflated with carbon dioxide. The intra-abdominal pressure is kept at about 15 mmHg, just enough to keep the anterior abdominal wall off the viscera. The Verres needle is then replaced by an 11 mm port site. A camera (rigid endoscope) is introduced through this port and three further ports are sited under direct vision — one is at the epigastrium and two further along the right costal margin, to allow the instruments and graspers access.

The gallbladder is retracted upwards, lifting up the liver and allowing the gallbladder bed to be visualised. The cystic artery and the cystic duct are ligated with clips and divided. Any adhesions between the gallbladder and surrounding structures are divided and the gallbladder is removed through the largest port hole (often placed in a plastic bag first). The gallbladder bed is washed and haemostasis is checked. The gas is removed and the peritoneum is closed with one or two sutures to the larger port holes.

Complications of Laparoscopic Cholecystectomy

General

The increased intra-abdominal pressure when the pneumoperitoneum is created can lead to a decreased venous return and hence can cause strain to the heart and lungs. Rarely, a CO_2 embolism can occur, which causes the patient to become very unwell.

Specific

- Bleeding from the cystic or hepatic artery can be much more difficult to deal with laparoscopically.
- Common bile duct injury has a reported incidence that is much higher in laparoscopic cholecystectomy compared to the open operation. This may, however, decrease in the future as surgeons become more experienced with the technique.
- Instrumentation injury, for example thermocoagulation of tissues with diathermy.

Some laparoscopic operations are technically diifcult or encounter complications, and conversion to an open procedure needs to take place.

Before performing a cholecystectomy the surgeon must establish whether there are any stones in the bile ducts as well as in the gallbladder. There are likely to be stones in the bile duct if there the patient is jaundiced, if the LFT's are abnormal (especially raised alkaline phosphatase) or if the ultrasound shows dilated bile ducts. If there are stones present in the bile ducts, then there is a choice between doing an ERCP before the operation (to remove the stones or perform a sphincterotomy) and doing an on-table cholangiogram and some form of bile duct exploration (either open or laparoscopic). The best management of bile duct stones in the new laparoscopic era is still not clear and results of clinical trials are awaited.

GALLSTONE ILEUS

Gallstone ileus is a misnomer; it is a small bowel obstruction and not an ileus (an ileus is a condition where there is absence of peristalsis in the intestine such as usually occurs for a few days after a laparotomy). It is relatively rare but is frequently asked about in finals.

In the normal anatomical position the gallbladder lies adjacent to the duodenum. A gallstone ileus is caused when a large gallstone (usually >2.5 cm) erodes directly through the wall of the gallbladder into the duodenum. Small gallstones will not cause obstruction, and they normally enter the duodenum by passing down the cystic duct and then the common bile duct. The erosion of a large gallstone directly into the duodenum is a process which probably occurs over a very long period of time. Surrounding inflammation seals the area such that no local abscess or peritonitis occurs in these cases. Once in the dudoenum the stone starts to be moved down the intestine by peristalsis. The narrowest part of the intestinal tract (after the gastro-oesophageal junction) is about 2 feet proximal to the ileocaecal valve and it is here that the gallstone may impact. The classical X-ray would show the signs of distal small bowel obstruction, air within the biliary tree (because of the fistula between the gallbladder and the duodenum) and the gallstone in the right lower quadrant of the abdomen. However, most cases are not diagnosed until surgery. Treatment is removal of the stone through an enterotomy (incision in the small bowel). The gallbladder is usually left alone, as removal can lead to a hole in the duodenum.

MUCOCOELE

A mucocoele is a condition where the drainage of the gallbladder is blocked by a stone which becomes impacted in the cystic duct. Mucus secreted by the gallbladder wall then builds up and gradually distends the gallbladder. Because this occurs slowly the gallbladder can reach a large size. A mucocoele may be completely asymptomatic or may present as a mass in the right upper quadrant. If it becomes infected an abscess can form ("infected mucocoele").

CHOLANGITIS

Cholangitis is a condition where there is infection within the biliary tree, and it is rare unless there is associated obstruction of the biliary tree. This a demonstration of the surgical principle that obstructed tubes tend to get infected (i.e. appendicitis, pyelonephritis, etc.). Cholangitis is clinically manifested by Charcot's triad of pain, jaundice and rigors (involuntary shivering attacks in association with a pyrexia). It requires prompt diagnosis and treatment, otherwise it can have a high mortality. Treatment consists of resuscitaton with fluids and the administration of intravenous antibiotics. If resolution is not rapid then attempts to produce biliary drainge, either endoscopically, radiologically or surgically, are required.

CARCINOMA OF THE GALLBLADDER

This is relatively rare and highly malignant. Unfortunately most cases are incurable at the time of presentation. It is associated with long-standing gallstones, polyps of the gallbladder (if a gallbladder polyp is >1 cm in size, then a cholecystectomy should probably be performed) and calcification of the gallbladder (known as a "porcelain" gallbladder), which is also an indication for cholecystectomy.

CARCINOMA OF THE PANCREAS

Adenocarcinoma of the pancreas is highly malignant and has usually metastasised by the time of diagnosis. It is rare before the age of 40 and is more common in smokers, diabetics and alcoholics. 60% of cases occur in the head, 25% in the body and 15% in the tail. It may present with obstructive jaundice, abdominal pain (which may radiate into the back), weight loss, anorexia, malaise or, rarely, thrombophlebitis migrans, although classically if you see an elderly patient with painless obstructive jaundice this would probably be top of your list. On examination there may be a mass or lymphadenopathy, hepatomegaly or ascites. The gallbladder may be palpable. Courvoisier's law states that if, in the presence of jaundice, the gallbladder is palpable, then the cause is unlikely to be gallstones.

Investigations include basic blood tests and specific diagnosis by ultrasound, CT or MRI. The ERCP may be helpful too, and may also allow therapeutic manoeuvres such as stent insertion (see section on obstructive jaundice).

Most tumours are treated palliatively (which may involve a bypass procedure); only a very small number are suitable for curative surgery (Whipple's operation — see Fig. 5.1). Five-year survival is very poor (<10%).

PANCREATITIS

The pathology of pancreatitis is that pancreatic enzyme precursors are released and activated, leading to a vicious circle of events. The exact mechanism for this is unknown but the end result is that the activated enzymes autodigest the pancreas. There are four stages to the process and resolution can occur at any point in the sequence of events. Initially there is oedema and fluid shifts which can lead to severe hypovolaemic shock (the patient is also vomiting, which compounds fluid losses). Fluid and enzymes are released into the peritoneal cavity, which may lead to autodigestion of fats (which can mop up calcium-forming soaps; and the patient may develop hypocalcaemia over the subsequent days, which is one of the markers of severity).

The second stage occurs when the autodigestion affects the blood vessels and can lead to haemorrhage into the retroperitoneal space. This accounts for Grey Turner's sign (bruising in the flanks) and Cullen's sign (bruising in the peri-umbilical area), although these signs are rare as the patient would be extremely ill at this point and usually in intensive care.

The third stage occurs when there is infarction due to the damaged blood supply and the pancreas becomes necrotic. Finally, the necrotic tissue can become infected, leading to abscess formation.

Acute pancreatitis usually presents with acute onset abdominal pain usually associated with raised levels of pancreatic amylase in the blood and urine. Recurrent attacks may occur, which are termed "relapsing acute pancreatitis". Chronic panreatitis is a different condition, where there is continuing inflammation and damage to the pancreas over a prolonged period of time, gradually associated with irreversible loss of function and pancreatic calcification and fibrosis. There are many factors capable of initiating an acute pancreatitis, although gallstones (these account for more than 50%) and alcohol abuse are the commonest. The mnemonic GET SMASH'N is often used by students — Gallstones, Ethanol, Trauma, Steroids (and other drugs such as azathioprine), Mumps (viral infections, including coxsackie B), Autoimmune diseases (e.g. SLE), Scorpion bites (rare and not in the UK), Hyperlipaemia (and hyperparathyroidism and hypothermia) and Neoplasia. All of these should be asked about in the history, especially alcohol intake.

A patient with acute pancreatitis will usually present with a sudden onset of severe upper abdominal or epigastric pain which may radiate directly through to the back. The patient may also have nausea or vomiting and the condition may rapidly progress to involve the whole abdomen and lead to shock. Usually the abdomen is diffusely tender but soft with normal bowel sounds; however, with significant acute pancreatitis the abdomen can have an appearance similar to peritonitis with the patient preferring to lie still, with widespread guarding and rigidity and absent bowel sounds.

There is no absolute test for a diagnosis of pancreatitis. The condition should be suspected in cases with the above presentation, but sometimes it can be impossible to exclude other causes of the acute abdomen, such as a perforated ulcer, without recourse to laparotomy.

The most useful test is the serum amylase level, but this can be normal in up to 30% of patients. If serum amylase is greater than 1200 IU this is usually diagnostic of pancreatitis; however, the degree of elevation of the serum amylase does not bear any clear relationship to the severity of the pancreatitis. If it is available a CT scan with intravenous contrast can be helpful in showing a swollen pancreas or pancreatic necrosis in severe cases.

Most units carry out something called "Ranson's criteria" in order to attempt to categorise pancreatitis into degrees of severity (see table). The blood tests that should be done are therefore those used in Ranson's scoring, namely a full blood count, U & E's, glucose, LFT's, calcium and arterial blood gases. An erect chest X-ray and an abdominal X-ray are performed. The erect CXR is for several reasons most important in helping to rule out the differential diagnosis of a perforated peptic ulcer (free air under the diaphragm), but also because the patient can get respiratory complications such as ARDS.

The aims of treatment are resuscitation of the patient with intravenous fluids and oxygen, analgesia and resting of the pancreas. Thus the patient is kept nil by mouth and a nasogastric tube is inserted to remove any gastric juices that may stimulate the pancreas. Fluid balance charts must be kept and a urinary catheter is needed to accurately monitor hourly urine output. Large fluid volumes may need to be given, the aim being to maintain a urine output of greater than 30 ml/h.

There is still debate about the precise role of antibiotics in acute pancreatitis, but most units do not routinely give antibiotics (except for cases of severe pancreatitis with Ranson's score greater than 4). Similarly, there is debate about the role of H2 blockers, although some units do give them routinely to all patients with pancreatitis.

Pethidine is the analgesic that is usually necessary for the pain of patients. Once on the ward they are carefully monitored and usually they settle with conservative treatment (checking the drug chart to see how much of the analgesic has been required is a good way of seeing if the pain is settling). If you look at the fluid balance you can see how much fluid has been sequestered into the abdominal cavity. On the ward round the consultant usually will request an investigation to look for the cause. This is usually an ultrasound first to look for gallstones (if gallstones are found, then the patient will need an elective cholecystectomy in the future to remove the cause).

The complications of acute pancreatitis include severe progressive shock leading to multiorgan failure and respiratory failure with an ARDS type picture. Pancreatic necrosis may become infected, forming a pancreatic abscess. This can be diagnosed by CT-guided aspiration of nonenhancing areas seen on a contrast-enhanced CT scan. If infected pancreatic necrosis is present, pancreatic debridement at laparotomy is indicated, although this operation has a high mortality. Such pancreatic abscesses are in fact the commonest cause of death in acute pancreatitis. Overall the mortality rate in acute pancreatitis is 10%. One other complication is a pancreatic pseudocyst which is a collection of fluid in the lesser sac (the space behind the stomach and lesser omentum in front of the pancreas). Diagnosis is usually by ultrasound in a patient who may have an epigastric mass or a swinging fever and a persistently elevated white cell count. In the first few weeks some cysts may reabsorb spontaneously, but if they persist they may need drainage either under radiological control or surgically. The traditional operation is to drain the cyst into the posterior wall of the stomach (cystogastrostomy).

Ranson's criteria for acute pancreatitis

One point for each variable. A score of 3 or more indicates severe pancreatitis.

1. *At Admission*
   (a) age greater than 55 years
   (b) blood glucose > 11 mmol/l
   (c) serum LDH > 500 IU/l
   (d) AST > 200 IU/l
   (e) white blood count > 16×10^9/l

(contd.)

2. *At 48 h After Admission*
   (a) haematocrit fall > 10%
   (b) blood urea > 16 mmol/l
   (c) serum calcium < 2 mmol/l
   (d) arterial pO_2 < 8 kPa
   (e) base deficit < 4 mmol/l

OBSTRUCTIVE JAUNDICE

Jaundice can be classified in several ways. The most common is to divide it into prehepatic (such as is caused by haemolytic anaemia), hepatic (caused by hepatitis) and posthepatic jaundice (which is also called obstructive jaundice or, sometimes, surgical jaundice). Prehepatic and hepatic causes of jaundice are usually dealt with as medical conditions not requiring surgery and will not be referred to further in this chapter. An additional type of obstructive jaundice should, however, be mentioned, namely drug-induced cholestatic jaundice, which is produced by drugs such as chlorpromazine. Clinically and biochemically this can be impossible to differentiate from true obstructive jaundice without further tests, and it is important that all cases of jaundice have a careful drug history taken.

The classical symptoms of obstructive jaundice are, first of all, the yellow appearance of the skin and mucous membranes. Quite often patients will have had this pointed out to them by a friend or relative rather than noticing it themselves. In addition they may have noticed a change in their urine and stools, with the urine becoming darker and the stools becoming paler. The urine becomes darker because conjugated bilirubin appears in it and the stool becomes paler because no bilirubin is entering the bowel. In addition the patient may complain of itching, which is caused by the deposition of bile salts in the skin (not bilirubin!). Pain is a variable feature in posthepatic obstructive jaundice. It is more common when jaundice is caused by gallstones. But it may still be a feature even with obstruction due to carcinoma at the head of the pancreas. These two entities, gallstones and carcinoma of the pancreas, are the main areas to be discussed when answering questions about obstructive jaundice in surgical finals, as they each constitute about one third of causes of obstructive jaundice (the other third are due to cholangiocarcinoma, chronic pancreatitis and enlarged lymph nodes in the porta hepatis).

Clinical Assessment

Clinical assessment in obstructive jaundice consists, first of all, of taking a full history. The importance in noting any drug therapy has been mentioned above. The duration of symptoms, associated weight loss (which can be particularly marked in obstructive jaundice, due to difficulty in fat and vitamin absorption), as well as the specific features of obstructive jaundice (itching, pale stools, dark urine), should be noted.

Physical examination will reveal jaundice itself. Jaundice is usually best seen by examining the sclerae of the eyes. Bilirubin levels above 50 µmol/l are usually clinically detectable (the normal range is up to 17 µmol/l). Other features to look for on physical examination include the stigmata of chronic liver disease (spider naevi, liver palms, Dupuytren's contracture, liver flap, gynaecomastia, testicular atrophy, etc.).

Examination of the abdomen should look for enlargement or tenderness of the liver and the presence of ascites. If the gallbladder is palpable, then Courvoisier's rule should be considered. This rule states that if in the presence of jaundice the gallbladder is palpable, then the cause of jaundice is unlikely to be stones. The reason for this rule is that when gallstones have been present for a significant period of time, chronic cholecystitis results in a thickening fibrosis of the gallbladder wall, making it unable to distend even when obstruction occurs. An exception is when there is dual pathology. A distended gallbladder will be felt underneath the right costal margin as a smooth convex, perhaps slightly tender, mass which moves down with the liver with inspiration.

Basic investigations in patients with jaundice will include full blood count, urea and electrolytes, liver function tests, and a chest X-ray. The liver function tests will confirm the obstructive nature of the jaundice.

Bilirubin will be raised, but the specific liver enzyme that will be raised predominantly will be the alkaline phosphatase rather than the transaminases. In addition all jaundice patients should have their baseline clotting status checked. The next most important test is the ultrasound scan, which is a quick and cheap way of demonstrating whether there is extra hepatic biliary obstruction, whether gallstones are present and perhaps whether there is a tumour in the pancreas. Ultrasound is very good at determining dilation of the biliary tree and common bile duct (the normal maximum upper limit for the width of the common bile duct is 7 mm). Up to 1.1 cm in diameter may be normal if there was previous obstruction which has now resolved. A width of the common bile duct greater than 1.1 cm is always abnormal. Ultrasound is also very good at looking at the gallbladder and for the presence of gallstones. Unfortunately the lower end of the common bile duct and the head of the pancreas are often poorly seen on ultrasound, due to overlying bowel gas. This is a particular problem in an overweight patient. If further imaging is felt to be needed, then it will usually be carried out by the ERCP (endoscopic retrograde cholangiopancreaticogram) and perhaps a CT or MRI scan. The ERCP enables biopsy or cytology to be performed.

Nowadays the mainstay of treatment in obstructive jaundice is either endoscopy (i.e. the ERCP) or, sometimes, endoscopy combined with subsequent surgery. The options are probably best illustrated by describing certain clinical examples:

Example 1: Obstructive Jaundice Due to a Gallstone in the Common Bile Duct

In this situation the traditional surgical approach would have been to carry out an open cholecystectomy and exploration of the common bile duct. The common bile duct would have been opened longitudinally between stay sutures and the stone removed, perhaps using special instruments such as balloon catheters or Des Jardin's forceps. The bile duct would then have been closed over a T-tube which would have been brought out through the abdominal wall and connected to a drainage bag. The purpose of the T-tube is to allow decompression of the bile duct whilst the healing process is continued so that there is no buildup of biliary pressure, which might cause a bile leak and peritonitis. Between 8 and 10 days postoperatively an X-ray would have been done by injecting contrast down the T-tube to outline the biliary tree (this is called a T-tube cholangiogram). As long as there are no leaks and no residual stones it is safe to remove the T-tube (the tract left behind quickly closes off). Although this procedure is not common practice nowadays, these technical details are still sometimes asked about in exams.

Nowadays most units would consider relief of the obstruction by arranging for an ERCP and extraction of the stone endoscopically from the common bile duct using a stone grasping basket (Dormia basket). This is usually combined with a sphincterotomy (cutting) of the sphincter of Oddi at the lower end of the bile duct to enable passage of the stone. The ERCP is associated with a lower incidence of complications than open exploration of the bile duct. The principal complications are pancreatitis in approximately 1% of patients and bleeding in a further 1%. Cholangitis (see below) is not a major problem except when residual obstruction is left behind. In about 10% of patients the ERCP in unsuccessful, as the common bile duct cannot be cannulated. Surgery will then be needed.

Once the obstruction has been relieved the patient can be booked for a cholecystectomy.

Example 2: Obstructive Jaundice Due to a Carcinoma of the Pancreas in an Elderly Patient

In an unresectable cancer of the head of the pancreas or in an elderly patient with carcinoma of the pancreas, a procedure to bypass the obstruction is often performed. This can be achieved by the insertion of a biliary stent during the ERCP. Occasionally it may be difficult to pass the stent using this technique and an alternative approach is to pass a stent using a percutaneous approach to the dilated biliary system through the skin directly into the liver under radiological control. If it is impossible to intubate the obstruction using these techniques, then surgical intervention may be considered, which would usually be a biliary bypass procedure (Fig. 5.2). The prognosis of carcinoma of the pancreas is appalling and the vast majority will be dead within a year.

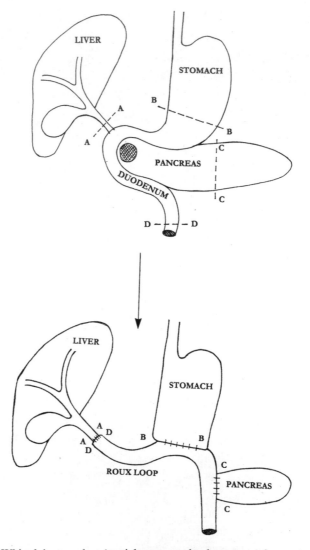

Figure 5.1. Whipple's procedure (partial pancreatoduodenectomy) for carcinoma of the head of the pancreas (shaded).

Example 3: Patients with Obstructive Jaundice Due to a Small Tumour with No Evidence of Metastatic Spread Who Are Relatively Young (Less Than 70 Years of Age)

This type of patient is relatively rare and may be considered for a Whipple operation. This operation involves excision of the head of the pancreas with the duodenum and therefore involves division of the bile duct and the pancreatic duct. Sometimes it is combined with partial gastrectomy, but most surgeons who perform these procedures nowadays do not remove the stomach and use the so-called "pylorus-preserving" technique. This is a major operation which can take 4–6 h, but it is the only procedure which offers any chance of cure for carcinoma of the pancreas. It should, however, only be used in patients where a cure is possible, and therefore those with tumours greater than 3 cm, or tumours fixed to the portal vein, and those in which metastases have already occurred should not be considered for this operation but should have some form of palliative procedure instead.

Example 4: Patients in Whom Insertion of an Endoscopic or Radiological Stent Is Impossible, or Patients in Whom an Endoscopic Stent Is Repeatedly Becoming Blocked

The major problem with biliary stents is blockage. This is thought to be due to deposition of bacterial by-products on the inside of the stent. To date there has been no good way of stopping this and the majority of stents will be blocked 3–6 months after insertion. Replacement of the stent is, however, usually a relatively simple procedure and thus stenting is still the treatment of choice in most patients with carcinoma of the pancreas because of their appallingly poor life expectancy. Occasionally, however, there may be patients in which a stent cannot be passed or is being blocked repeatedly, and if the patient is fit enough a palliative biliary bypass might be considered. This is usually carried out as a bypass either between the gallbladder or (preferably) the bile duct itself and the small bowel. Most surgeons prefer to construct a Roux loop for anastomosis of the gallbladder. If there is significant duodenal

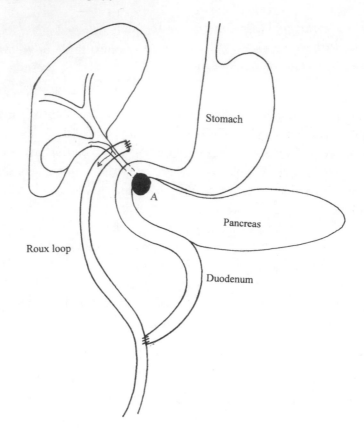

Figure 5.2. Biliary bypass with Roux loop (A = carcinoma in head of pancreas).

involvement, then gastric outflow obstruction may also be considered a problem and the biliary bypass may be combined with a gastric bypass operation. It must be stressed, however, that these procedures should be reserved for a small subgroup of patients with carcinoma of the pancreas where endoscopic therapy is not appropriate.

Specific Complications of Surgery in Jaundiced Patients

(1) *Coagulopathy.* Jaundiced patients often have impaired clotting. This is largely a failure to absorb vitamin K (one of the fat-soluble

vitamins) from the gut. This is manifested as a prolonged INR. It can be reversed by the intramuscular administration of vitamin K preoperatively. Other clotting problems may also be present, and a careful coagulation profile should be done on a jaundiced patient who is undergoing surgery and clotting factors such as fresh frozen plasma should be arranged as necessary.

(2) *Renal failure (hepatorenal syndrome)*. Patients with obstructive jaundice are much more prone to develop renal failure than patients undergoing similar degrees of surgery for other causes. The precise mechanisms underlying this are not well understood. The absorption of an endotoxin from the intestine (translocation) which is normally removed by the reticuloendothelium system of the liver, may be one factor. Additionally there may be some as yet unidentified factor produced by the liver itself which helps modulate renal function. In order to overcome this risk, jaundiced patients undergoing surgery should be fully hydrated preoperatively. This will mean their having an intravenous infusion set up the day before. In addition osmotic diuretics such as mannitol may be given during and after the procedure and dopamine infusion at 2.5 mcg/kg per min may also be given via a central line in order to maximize renal function. The patient may have a central line inserted to monitor the central venous pressure and a catheter to monitor hourly urine output, which should be kept at 40 ml per hour or greater.

(3) *Nutrition*. Patients with obstruction especially due to carcinoma are often very malnourished. There may be a history of marked weight loss. These patients may need nutritional support pre- or postoperatively. The most important factor is, however, to overcome the obstruction. There is no evidence that prolonged intravenous nutrition preoperatively is an advantage in these patients.

(4) *Infection*. Patients with obstructive jaundice appear to have a greater incidence of infection problems including wound complications. This may be partly due to their poor protein status and there is a nonspecific effect of malignancy on the immune system. The patient should be appropriately covered with broad spectrum antibiotics, preferably those which appear in the bile.

(5) *Cholangitis.* Cholangitis is one of the most-feared complications in obstructive jaundice. It is the cause of Charcot's triad, which consists of rigors or fever, abdominal pain and jaundice. It is caused by infection within an obstructed biliary tree. It should be regarded as an emergency, as left untreated it can result in severe shock, renal failure and death.

6

OESOPHAGUS, STOMACH AND DUODENUM

Disorders of the oesophagus, stomach and duodenum are mainly dealt with by gastroenterologists. It is the aspects of these disorders which relate to surgery which are discussed here. Most of these conditions give rise to symptoms rather than signs, and upper gastrointestinal endoscopy is the mainstay of diagnosis. In finals, questions about these conditions are most likely to appear in the written, viva or long case section of the exam. Short cases relating to the conditions will be relatively rare.

DYSPHAGIA

Dysphagia is a symptom. It means difficulty in swallowing, and not pain on swallowing. Most disorders of the oesophagus that are of relevance to the surgical finals examination have dysphagia as a pre-senting symptom. Some of the disorders which can cause dysphagia are shown in the following table, with a useful way of subclassifying them.

Causes of Dysphagia

---

1. *In the lumen*

   • Foreign bodies (especially in children and psychiatric patients)
   • Polypoid tumours

(contd.)

2. *In the wall*

    - Benign strictures (usually associated with reflux oesophagitis, or occasionally ingestion of caustic substances)
    - Malignant strictures
    - Achalasia
    - Oesophageal web (Plummer–Vinson syndrome; usually middle-aged women with iron deficiency anaemia — the webs consist of desquamated epithelium)
    - Scleroderma
    - Candidiasis

3. *Outside the wall (extrinsic compression from)*

    - Pharyngeal pouch
    - Rolling hiatus hernia
    - Malignancy
    - Retrosternal goitre
    - Vascular structures such as thoracic aortic aneurysms or congenitally abnormal vessels (dysphagia lusoria)

4. *Systemic causes*

    - Myasthenia gravis
    - Pseudobulbar palsy
    - Hysteria

OESOPHAGEAL CANCER

Oesophageal cancer is relatively uncommon but is unfortunately highly malignant. The oesophagus is normally lined by squamous epithelium but there may be some gastric type mucosa at its lower end. Carcinoma of the oesophagus may therefore either be squamous (95%) or adenocarcinoma (5%). 15% of squamous carcinomas occur in the upper third, 50% in the middle third and 35% in the lower third. Adenocarcinoma usually occurs at the lower end of the oesophagus.

Barrett's oesophagus is a condition where the normal squamous epithelium in the distal oesophagus is replaced with glandular epithelium. It is thought to be caused by chronic gastro-oesophageal reflux of acid. Its major clinical significance is that patients have an increased risk of developing adenocarcinoma of the oesophagus. Other risk factors are smoking, alcohol, and nitrosamine intake in food (which may explain its high incidence in certain parts of the world, e.g. South Africa).

Most oesophageal cancers present with dysphagia, by which time spread has often occurred. Without treatment the average survival from diagnosis is nine months. Staging is using the TNM method (i.e. Tumour, Node, Metastases — see page 180). Dysphagia is usually first for solids and then for liquids (as one might expect) and is usually progressive. Patients will often have altered their eating habits to take more liquid and softer foods in the earlier stages and weight loss is common at presentation. Aspiration pneumonia may also be present as a result of overflow obstruction, particularly at night (i.e. food/fluid in the oesophagus tracks back up and trickle down into the airways). Physical examination may show lymphadenopathy or hepatomegaly and ascites etc., but often there will be no abnormalities on examination other than obvious weight loss. The mainstay of investigation is either endoscopy or barium swallow. The typical appearance on barium swallow is of a "shouldered" stricture rather the smoother tapered narrowing seen with a benign stricture. Endoscopy offers the additional advantage of allowing biopsy or cytology to confirm the diagnosis. CT scanning or magnetic resonance scanning may be helpful in assessing the degree of spread and invasion of adjacent structures and whether the tumour is surgically resectable. Endoscopic ultrasound (a special ultrasound probe which goes down the endoscope) is a relatively new development which is becoming increasingly used to assess invasion and help predict resectability.

The aim of treatment in carcinoma of the oesophagus is to cure where possible and palliate where not. Surgery, where feasible, offers the greatest opportunity for cure. However, probably only 50–60% of patients have a technically resectable tumour at presentation, and even in those where the tumour is technically resectable, micrometastatic spread will often have occurred and cure will therefore not be a possibility. There are several surgical approaches to resection of the oesophagus. The principle of most of them is to resect the oesophagus and mobilize the stomach up so that it can be brought up into the chest or neck for anastomosis to the remaining oesophagus. To do this, incisions may be required abdominally, in the chest (thoracotomy) or in the neck. If inoperable then radiotherapy may be helpful but only for squamous carcinoma (squamous carcinomas generally tend to be much more sensitive to radiotherapy than adenocarcinomas). Where the tumour is inoperable, dysphagia may be relieved by insertion of a plastic or metal tube (stent), usually at endoscopy. Unfortunately, these often block off either because of tumour infiltration or by food getting stuck in the lumen (fizzy drinks may help). Sometimes a laser is used to temporarily relieve dysphagia. The overall five-year survival rate for carcinoma of the oesophagus is 10–15%.

PHARYNGEAL POUCH

A pharyngeal pouch (also known as Zenker's diverticulum) is an out-pouching of the pharynx, usually between the upper border of the cricopharyngeous muscle and the lower border of the inferior constrictor muscle of the pharynx — through a weak area called Kilian's dehiscence. It is thought to be a so-called "pulsion" diverticulum, i.e. it is caused by peristaltic activity pumping against resistance due to discoordinate muscle spasm. Although it comes out posteriorly, it usually appears on the left side of the neck and may produce a palpable lump on neck examination. On eating, food enters the diverticulum, which then expands and presses on the adjacent oesophagus, causing the dysphagia. Patients may also complain of regurgitation of food from the diverticulum, gurgling sounds, or bad breath because of the presence of decaying food in the diverticulum. Sometimes a patient will learn to make the pouch empty by using external pressure on the neck. One complication of the oesophageal pouch is perforation at endoscopy when the endoscope enters the pouch instead of continuing down the oesophagus, and pressure on the scope to try and make it pass further causes a perforation. Treatment is either by excision of the pouch or an operation to invert it into the lumen. Sometimes a myotomy (division of muscle fibres of cricopharyngeous muscle) is also carried out to relieve spasm.

PERFORATION OF THE OESOPHAGUS

Oesophageal perforation may be caused by trauma at endoscopy or from a sharp foreign body, such as a fish bone. Spontaneous rupture of the oesophagus (Boerhaave's syndrome) occurs with forceful or prolonged vomiting. The significance of perforation of the oesophagus is that it will usually lead to mediastinitis (infection and inflammation of the mediastinum as a result of food/fluid entering the mediastinum). This is a rapidly progressive and serious condition requiring prompt diagnosis and treatment if death of the patient is to be avoided. Treatment for anything but the most minor perforation would normally include surgery to repair or resect the oesophagus and wash out and drain the mediastinum along with appropriate resuscitation and antibiotics.

REFLUX DISEASE AND HIATUS HERNIA

The oesophagus passes into the abdomen from the thorax through the oesophageal hiatus of the diaphragm. Normally about 2–4 cm of the oesophagus lies within the abdomen. Hiatus hernias may either be rolling (10%), sliding (85%) or mixed (5%). In rolling hiatus hernia the junction between the lower end of the oesophagus and the stomach (the cardio-oesophageal junction) is in the normal position and the hernia is caused by the stomach rolling up beside the oesophagus. In sliding hiatus hernia the oesophagogastric junction moves up into the thorax.

Hiatus hernia commonly presents with retrosternal burning pains, which may be worse on bending, stooping or at night in bed. Such symptoms are often called heartburn by patients, who may also report regurgitation of acid fluid into their mouth. Patients will normally report that the pain is worse after meals and will usually have noticed that they

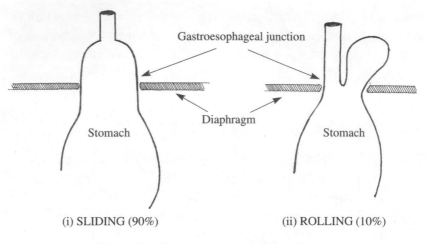

Figure 6.1. The two main types of hiatus hernia.

get at least some relief by proprietary antacids. Severe reflux oesophagitis may lead to ulceration and bleeding or, if long-standing, benign stricture formation. Treatment of hiatus hernia involves measures such as losing weight, stoping smoking, eating smaller meals, etc. Antacids, H2 receptor antagonists and drugs which mechanically prevent reflux by forming a raft on top of the stomach, such as some of the alginate preparations, may be helpful. For significant oesphagitis, however, one of the newer proton pump inhibitors is probably the drug of choice. Where medical therapy has failed or where the patient is unhappy with the prospect of permanent medication, surgery may be indicated. Many operations have been described but the commonest one is Nissen's fundoplication, which involves mobilising the fundus of the stomach and wrapping it around the lower end of the oesophagus in order to provide a new sphincter mechanism to prevent reflux. This operation is often performed laparoscopically nowadays.

ACHALASIA OF THE OESOPHAGUS

This is due to failure of relaxation of the smooth muscle at the lower end of the oesophagus due to an abnormality of its nerve supply. It usually presents in middle life and the precise cause is unknown. It has some similarities to the tropical disease trypanosomiasis (Chagas' disease), in which the nerve supply to the oesophageal muscle is also deficient. It usually presents with intermittent dysphagia with a gradual progression. Unlike dysphagia in carcinoma of the oesophagus, the symptoms are usually worse for liquids than for solids. The patient may also complain of fluid regurgitation, which may be worse at night and associated with pneumonia. The diagnosis is usually made on barium swallow and the typical features are of a dilated oesophagus above a smooth tapering stricture, sometimes called a "rat tail stricture", and the absence of a gastric air bubble on a plain X-ray (carcinoma of the oesophagus normally develops too rapidly to allow significant oesophageal dilatation, whereas in achalasia the gradual development of the condition may lead to the oesophagus being enormous above). Achalasia is treated either by dilatation under X-ray control or by an operation called Heller's procedure. Heller's procedure is a cardiomyotomy, i.e. an operation which involves dividing the muscle layer at the lower end of the oesophagus (the cardia) down as far as the mucosa. The mucosa is left intact. This operation is similar in principle to Ramstedt's operation for infantile hypertrophic pyloric stenosis. Squamous carcinoma of the oesophagus develops in 3–5% of patients with achalasia.

PEPTIC ULCERATION

Peptic ulcers are defined as ulcers caused by acid and can occur at several sites, namely the duodenum (commonest), the stomach, the oesophagus, the jejunum (in Zollinger–Ellison syndrome — see page 113), Meckel's diverticulum (if it contains ectopic gastric mucosa) and sometimes at the site of a gastroenterostomy

Obviously duodenal and stomach ulcers form the vast majority of those cases seen clinically, but in an essay answer it is important to be able discuss these other areas at least in broad outline.

Likewise, the complications that a peptic ulcer, at any site, can produce can be listed as:

- Pain
- Bleeding (acute or chronic)
- Penetration into adjacent structures (into the pancreas for a posterior duodenal ulcer)
- Perforation (usually an anterior duodenal or gastric ulcer)
- Obstruction (i.e. severe scarring of the pylorus from chronic ulceration or acute obstruction of the pylorus from acute ulceration with oedema)
- Pancreatitis (rare)
- Biliary obstruction (rare)

DUODENAL ULCERATION

Duodenal ulceration occurs more frequently in men than in women and has a peak in the age group between 45 and 55 years of age. 95% of duodenal ulceration is within the first part of the duodenum, within 2 cm of the pylorus. Patients often describe pain as being eased by food (unlike gastric ulcers, where it is often worsened by food), and it is often worse at night and may radiate through to the back. Nowadays the treatment is usually medical. Attention should be paid to getting the patient to stop smoking, and if he is on any drugs such as nonsteroidal anti-inflammatory drugs or aspirin, they should be stopped. It is very important that new symptoms in any patient over the age of 35 are investigated with a gastroscopy to make sure that the problem is simple benign ulceration and not the early presentation of a gastric carcinoma. In addition biopsies can be taken for *Helicobacter pylori* identification. Treatment would normally consist of an H2 antagonist or proton pump inhibitor in combination with antibiotics to eradicate *Helicobacter* where indicated. With this regime the majority of duodenal ulcers can be medically managed and relatively few will come to surgery.

GASTRIC ULCERS

Gastric ulceration has a different peak age to duodenal ulceration and occurs maximally between 55 and 65 years of age. As gastric ulcers can sometimes be malignant, all patients greater than 35 years of age with indigestion need to be carefully investigated (by biopsy) to exclude this. As with duodenal ulceration, the treatment is mainly medical. Surgery is rarely required.

GASTRIC AND DUODENAL ULCER SURGERY

In the surgical exam, in-depth knowledge of gastric physiology will not be required. The following principles are, however, important. Firstly, without any acid there can be no ulcer and, in broad terms, whether or not an ulcer develops is the result of the balance between acid secretion and the mucosal protective factors which are reduced by drugs such as nonsteroidal anti-inflammatory drugs. Remember that the stomach starts at the oesophagogastric junction (called the cardia). There is a fundus, a body and an antrum that leads through the pylorus into the duodenum (the fundus and body contain cells that produce the acid, pepsinogen and intrinsic factor, whereas the major site of gastrin formation is in the antrum). Most peptic ulceration is in the first part of the duodenum but may spread further down and even be found in the small bowel in Zollinger–Ellison syndrome (see page 113). Gastric acid secretion is stimulated by either gastrin or vagal nerve stimulation. There are two vagus nerves supplying the stomach, i.e. the right and the left vagus, which actually sit in a posterior and an anterior position close to the oesophagus as it enters the abdomen. Smaller divisions of these vagus nerves, called the nerves of Latarjet, supply the pyloric region and are responsible for relaxation of the pylorus to allow emptying of the stomach. Other branches of the nerves supply the acid-secreting areas of the stomach. This explains why a truncal vagotomy (division of the vagus nerves as they enter the abdomen) results in reduced acid secretion, but a stomach which fails to empty adequately. A truncal vagotomy operation, therefore, needs to be combined with a further procedure to enable emptying of the stomach, such as a gastroenterostomy or a pyloroplasty.

As stated above, these operations are now rarely required for elective peptic ulcers. Questions are, however, often asked about them in surgical finals, but you will be expected to know only the principles of the common operations, not technical details.

VAGOTOMY

Because the vagus nerves supply the stomach and stimulate the release of acid, division of these nerves can reduce the amount of acid produced. A vagotomy may either be truncal, selective or highly selective. A truncal vagotomy is where the vagi are divided as they enter the abdomen. The problem with truncal vagotomy is that the nerves required to relax the pyloric muscle and produce pyloric opening are also divided and a truncal vagotomy, therefore, usually has to be combined with a so-called "drainage procedure", such as a pyloroplasty or gastroenterostomy. Other types of vagotomy include selective or highly selective vagotomies. The principle of these operations is to leave intact the nerve supply to the pylorus (Latarjet) while dividing the branches to the rest of the stomach so that the acid secretion is suppressed but pyloric emptying is maintained.

DRAINAGE PROCEDURES

The two commonest drainage procedures are pyloroplasty and gastroenterostomy.

A *pyloroplasty* is a procedure by which an incision is made across the pylorus from the distal stomach into the proximal duodenum. The longitudinal incision is then closed transversely so as to widen the pylorus and to allow free emptying of the stomach. Do not confuse this procedure with a pyloromyotomy (Ramstedt's procedure — see page 117), where only the muscular layer is cut.

A *gastroenterostomy* is a procedure whereby a loop of proximal small bowel is brought up and anastomosed to the stomach. The small bowel can be brought up either behind the transverse colon (i.e. retrocolic) or in front of the transverse colon (i.e. anticolic). The stomach can then empty directly into the small bowel even if the pylorus will not open.

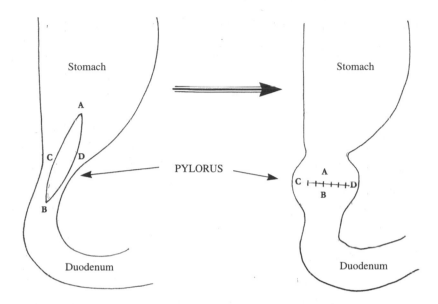

Figure 6.2. Pyloroplasty. A longitudinal incision (A–B) is made through the pylorus and then closed transversely (C–D) to widen it.

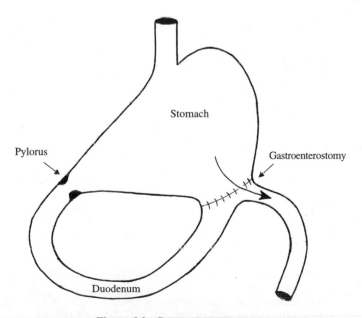

Figure 6.3. Gastroenterostomy.

ANTRECTOMY AND VAGOTOMY

In this operation the distal half of the stomach is removed (i.e. a partial gastrectomy) in combination with a truncal vagotomy procedure. The stomach can then be reanastomosed either directly to the duodenum

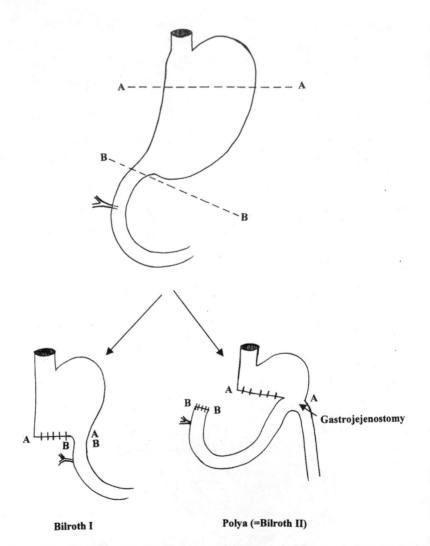

Bilroth I   **Polya (=Bilroth II)**

Figure 6.4. Gastrectomies. The distal part of the stomach (between A–A and B–B) is removed and the two main techniques for joining it up again are shown.

(Bilroth I procedure) or a duodenal stump can be closed over and a small bowel loop brought up for ananastomosis on to the stomach (Bilroth II procedure, also known as a Polya gastrectomy). The gallbladder remains attached to the second part of the duodenum.

NEAR TOTAL OR TOTAL GASTRECTOMY

This serious operation is nowadays never done for benign peptic ulceration, except occasionally where Zollinger–Ellison syndrome is present and cannot be treated medically. Its main role is in complete gastrectomy for carcinoma of the stomach. After total gastrectomy, intestinal continuity is usually reconstructed using a "Roux loop" of small bowel.

COMPLICATIONS OF PEPTIC ULCER SURGERY

Although peptic ulcer surgery is nowadays rarely performed, the complications are specific and sometimes asked about in final exams. The following shows a way of classifying them. Remember that complications can be general and specific, etc. The following shows in detail only the specific complications related to the peptic ulcer operations, (also see page 34).

Early Complications

- *Haemorrhage*
- *Duodenal stump leakage*
- Failure of the stomach to empty and *bilious vomiting* (occurs in 10% of patients)

Late Complications

- *Postvagotomy diarrhoea*
- *Afferent loop syndrome* (i.e. problems because of a long blind-ended

bowel loop as left in a Bilroth II gastrectomy — it causes either vomiting of bile or proliferation of bacteria leading to anaemia and malnutrition as in a blind loop syndrome.

- *Dumping syndrome* — characterised by abdominal distension, flushes, sweating and nausea. Can be divided into early and late dumping. *Early dumping* occurs immediately after the meal and is due to food entering the small bowel too rapidly and drawing fluid into the bowel by osmosis producing fluid shifts and hypotension. *Late dumping* occurs 1–2 h after the meal and is due to reactive hypoglycaemia caused by the wave of insulin produced in response to the rapid delivery of food into the small intestine. The treatment involves reassurance that most cases settle with time, and trying small low carbohydrate meals.
- *Alkaline gastritis*
- *Anaemia* (can be due to a lack of the intrinsic factor, vitamin B_{12} and iron)
- *Osteomalacia due to lack of vitamin D and calcium*
- *Recurrent ulceration and malignancy*

ZOLLINGER–ELLISON SYNDROME

Zollinger–Ellison syndrome is a hypersecretion of gastric acid due to a gastrin-producing tumour (gastrinoma). Most of these gastrinomas are in the pancreas but can also occasionally be found in the duodenum, stomach or ovary. They are part of the so-called APUDomas of the multiple endocrine neoplasia type I group. 60% are malignant and the rest benign. They can be very small in size and difficult to find with investigations or at operation. The classic features of Zollinger–Ellison syndrome is refractory peptic ulceration, which may involve the whole duodenum and even small bowel. The diagnosis is made by the demonstration of high gastrin levels in the presence of high acid secretion and the secretin test may be helpful in making this diagnosis. Appropriate investigations include CT scanning, magnetic resonance imaging and angiography, which may be combined with venous blood sampling for gastrin levels. New investigations of interest include intraoperative ultrasound to look for small tumours in the pancreas. The treatment is essentially medical with drugs such as the proton pump inhibitors combined with surgery if the position of the tumour can be identified. Surgery has two roles: firstly, removal of the tumour; and secondly, carrying out antiulcer operations such as vagotomy or gastrectomy.

Multiple Endocrine Neoplasia (MEN)

MEN Type I

- Hyperparathyroidism (parathyroid hyperplasia)
- Insulinoma of pancreas
- Pituitary tumours
- Zollinger–Ellison syndrome (gastrinoma), adrenocortical tumours and carcinoid tumours

MEN Type II

Medullary cell carcinoma of thyroid and phaeochromacytoma plus others, depending on the type, IIa or IIb.

MEN II	IIa (Sipple's Syndrome)	IIb
Medullary cell carcinoma of thyroid and phaeochro-mocytoma plus	Hyperparathyroidism	"Marfanoid" habitus Submucosal neurofibromata of the tongue, eyelids and lips

UPPER GASTROINTESTINAL BLEEDING

This is a common topic in the exams and appears in both medical and surgical finals. It is important because it is one of the things that house officers will have to deal with and it is perceived as being a good way of sorting out those who know the basics about emergency care from those who do not. Overall upper gastrointestinal bleeding has a significant mortality of 5–10%. It may present as either the frank vomiting of blood (haematemesis), the vomiting of blood which has been altered by being in the stomach for a period of time in the presence of gastric acid (coffee ground vomiting), or the passage per rectum of blood which has travelled down from the upper gastrointestinal tract and been altered in the process (melaena).

The following is a list of the most important causes of upper GI bleeding (note that peptic ulcer disease accounts for nearly 70%):

- Dudoenal ulcer (30%)
- Gastric ulcer (20%)
- Acute erosions or gastritis (20%)
- Mallory–Weiss tear (at the lower end of the oesophagus due to powerful vomiting; <10%)
- Oesophageal varices (5%)
- Oesophagitis (5%)
- Cancer of the stomach or oesophagus

The management of someone with upper gastrointestinal bleeding includes a full history and examination. Appropriate investigations would be a full blood count, urea and electrolytes, a blood clotting screen, a chest X-ray and cross-matching of blood. Patients should have intravenous access sited, preferably with two large bore peripheral lines and possibly a central venous line and in addition a urinary catheter to monitor urine output. All patients should have early endoscopy to identify the site of bleeding, and nowadays it is sometimes possible to inject the ulcer at endoscopy to reduce the chance of further bleeding. High risk groups for mortality from upper gastrointestinal bleeding include those patients aged greater than 60 years, those shocked at presentation, and those with coexistent disease such as heart or chest problems.

Persistent bleeding requiring greater than approximately 5 units transfusion and rebleeding during the same admission are usually regarded as indications for urgent surgery. Surgery usually consists of opening the stomach or duodenum and under-running the bleeding vessel in order to prevent it bleeding further, and an antiulcer procedure such as a truncal vagotomy and pyloroplasty. Patients bleeding from oesophageal varices are usually treated with injection sclerotherapy at endoscopy as well as resuscitation. If this is insufficient to stop immediate bleeding, then a double balloon tube (the commonest sort is called a Sengstaken tube) is inserted. The two balloons are designed to be positioned in the stomach and oesophagus to tamponade the bleeding sites.

PERFORATED PEPTIC ULCER

The commonest site of peptic ulcer perforation is the duodenum. Usually the ulcer is anterior (if it is posterior it is more likely to either penetrate into the pancreas or erode the gastroduodenal artery and cause haemorrhage). Surprisingly, many patients who present with a perforated peptic ulcer have had little in the way of pre-existing symptoms of indigestion. If these are present, however, or if there is a previous history of peptic ulcer, it may make the diagnosis more obvious. Because the pathology essentially involves the release of gastric or duodenal fluid into the peritoneal cavity, the way in which patients present is perhaps predictable. They will usually report a sudden onset of epigastric pain and vomiting and will often display the features of peritonitis, preferring to lie still as movement makes the pain worse. On examination they will have tenderness either in the upper abdomen where leakage has been minimal or over the whole abdomen where it has been more severe. They may have a rigid tender abdomen with rebound tenderness and percussion tenderness and absent bowel sounds. An erect chest X-ray is the key investigation, as it may show air beneath the diaphragm (note that air under the diaphragm is best shown on an erect chest X-ray and not a plain abdominal X-ray — this is a common misconception among students). However, only 60–70% of cases show this initially. Essentially the diagnosis is usually made of a generalised peritonitis, with the most likely cause being a perforated peptic ulcer. A laparotomy is indicated and therefore the patient is then resuscitated and prepared for theatre. For a simple duodenal ulcer perforation, the operation usually consists of washing out the abdomen to remove contamination and then closing the repair with a piece of omentum which is sutured as a patch over the hole. For a gastric ulcer perforation it is usually advisable to excise the ulcer with a small ellipse of stomach and then close the defect using sutures. The reason for this is that up to one third of gastric ulcers may prove to be malignant and the excised ulcer should be sent for histology to exclude this. Occasionally, with a very large perforation or in a patient who has had previous peptic ulcer problems and who has perforated despite being on appropriate medical therapy, it may be necessary to proceed on to do additional surgery. This may be either a partial gastrectomy or a procedure such as truncal vagotomy to reduce peptic acid secretion, which would normally be combined with either a pyloroplasty or a gastroenterostomy.

HYPERTROPHIC PYLORIC STENOSIS OF INFANCY

This is a condition which affects approximately 1 in 350 live births. It is one of the few paediatric surgical conditions frequently asked about in surgical finals. It is more common in male infants than in female, and for some reason in first-borns. The typical history would be of a baby who feeds normally at first and then, 3–10 weeks postdelivery, starts to develop vomiting which may be projectile in nature. Diagnosis can be made by ultrasound or gastrograffin (water-soluble) meal, but the traditional approach to diagnosis is that of a test feed in which the infant is allowed to feed while the abdomen is palpated. A positive test will be when a so-called pyloric tumour ("tumour" in Greek means "swelling") is felt, which consists of the hypertrophied pyloric muscle contracting. The treatment is usually surgical, with a division of the muscle fibres down to the mucosa but leaving the mucosa intact, and the pylorus can then empty normally. This is known as Ramstedt's operation.

GASTRIC CANCER

Gastric cancer is highly malignant and is usually diagnosed late in this country, although in some countries such as Japan so-called early gastric cancers are more frequently found. In this country there is a 5–10% five-year survival. The risk factors are thought to be smoking, dietary factors (hot spicy foods) and the presence of previous gastric surgery or pernicious anaemia. It is thought that in a stomach with less acid than normal, bacteria may exist which produce carcinogens. A genetic factor is the association with blood group A. The typical presentation would be weight loss and anorexia, epigastric pain, nausea and vomiting, and at a later stage the signs of generalised malignancy with weight loss, etc. Abdominal examination may reveal a mass, a succussion splash (fluid sits in the stomach and can be heard splashing when the patient's abdomen is shaken), ascites or hepatomegaly. A left supraclavicular lymph node may also be palpable (Virchow's node); when present this is known as Trosier's sign. Another association is with acanthosis nigricans (pigmented warty axillary skin). The diagnosis can be made by either barium meal or endoscopy. Endoscopy is preferred, as it enables multiple biopsies for histology to be taken. A CT or ultrasound scan may be helpful in staging.

Treatment can be any of the following:

- *Surgical* — either curative or palliative. (Even if the tumour is incurable, surgery is still the treatment of choice as it offers the best palliation. Most patients should have a laparotomy for attempted resection or palliative bypass.)
- *Chemotherapy* — palliative only; low response.
- *Medical palliation*, i.e. the passage of plastic tubes to allow stomach emptying, etc.
- *Radiotherapy* is of no value.

Surgical treatment for resectable tumours usually consists of gastrectomy, either partial (usually a Polya type gastrectomy) or complete. In complete gastrectomy the intestine continuity is usually restored using a Roux loop of small bowel. If the tumour is unresectable then a palliative bypass can be constructed using a gastroenterostomy above the tumour.

Gastric cancer is often used as a classic model for the way in which tumours spread, namely:

- Spread within the wall of the organ leading to the so-called linitis plastica (also known as a leather bottle stomach).
- Local spread to adjacent structures, such as the pancreas.
- Lymphatic spread such as occurs with spread to local lymph nodes and nodes further afield.
- Transcoelomic spread, where the tumour seeds across the peritoneal cavity.
- Blood-borne spread such as occurs with lung metastases.

7

SMALL INTESTINE AND COLON

MECKEL'S DIVERTICULUM

Meckel's diverticulum is a remnant of the vitello intestinal duct, which normally disappears during embryological development. It is found in approximately 2% of the population and occurs approximately 2 feet proximal to the iliocaecal valve on the antimesenteric border (the border not attached to the mesentery) of the ileum. Some books suggest that it is usually 2 inches in length (hence 2, 2, 2), but in fact its length is very variable. Sometimes it extends as far as the back of the umbilicus on the anterior abdominal wall, and indeed occasionally it may even present as mucosa protruding at the umbilicus when there is a so-called vitello intestinal fistula. This protruding mucosa is sometimes referred to as a raspberry tumour.

Meckel's diverticulum is usually completely asymptomatic. It can, however, present with:

- A picture similar to appendicitis.
- Bleeding.
- Volvulus or intussusception.

If the Meckel's becomes inflamed, it can produce a clinical presentation very similar to acute appendicitis. If a patient is taken to theatre for an appendicectomy and the appendix is found to be normal, a Meckel's should always be looked for. Occasionally a Meckel's will contain ectopic gastric mucosa, which can cause bleeding and is in fact the commonest cause of major gastrointestinal bleeding in teenagers. A further complication that a Meckel's can cause is a volvulus of the intestine if it is tethered to the abdominal wall. Occasionally it may also form the apex of an intussusception. Very often the diagnosis of a Meckel's is made at laparotomy, but occasionally it may be possible to use a technetium scan in cases of intestinal bleeding which can reveal a Meckel's by targeting the gastric mucosa within it. Once Meckel's diverticulum is identified, the treatment is simple — surgical excision.

TUMOURS OF THE SMALL INTESTINE

Tumours of the small intestine are relatively rare, comprising less than 5% of all gastrointestinal tumours. Often an examiner tries to throw a student by asking about them. This is not because you are expected to know much about them but because it is a good question to ask to see if you can think and answer a question logically; for example, "Tell me about small bowel tumours."

Approach this sort of question as discussed in the chapter "Surgical Talk" as follows — small bowel tumours can be primary or secondary, benign or malignant.

Benign Tumours

These can arise from any of the elements of the bowel wall, such as:

- Lipomas (arise from fat).
- Leiomyomas (arise from smooth muscle).
- Neurofibromas (arise from nerves).
- Adenomas (arise from glandular mucosa).
- Adenomatous polyps of the small bowel may be premalignant (as in the colon). As with colonic adenomas, they may also be associated with polyposis syndromes and Peutz–Jegher's syndrome (pigmentation around the mouth and small bowel polyps). Benign tumours may either be found incidentally or present with bleeding or intussusception.

MALIGNANCY OF THE SMALL INTESTINE

Adenocarcinoma of the small intestine is occasionally seen and is believed in the majority of cases to arise from pre-existing adenomatous polyps (as in the colon).

Lymphomas may also occur in the small bowel.

Carcinoid tumours are of low grade malignancy and are believed to arise from neuroectodermal cells embryologically. The commonest site for these is the appendix, but they can occur anywhere throughout the gastrointestinal tract and are also found in the lung (bronchial carcinoids). These tumours release serotonin (5-HT) and kinins, which can cause symptoms if they get into the circulation. Normally these hormones are broken down by the liver in the first pass metabolism from the gut and so no symptoms occur. However, in the presence of metastases there is no first pass metabolism and the patient may suffer from carcinoid syndrome which consisits of flushing, bronchospasm and diarrhoea.

INTUSSUSCEPTION

An intussusception can be defined as a condition where a portion of intestine gets invaginated (by peristalsis) into its own lumen. The invaginated portion (the intussusceptum) can then be further propelled down the lumen for a variable distance.

A section through a piece of bowel containing an intussusception would contain two full layers of intestinal wall: the intussusceptum inside and the intussuscipiens outside.

Most intussusceptions are seen in children, usually infants under one year of age. They may present as colicky abdominal pain leading to obstruction. So called redcurrant jelly stools may be passed (which consists of mucus and blood). The danger is that the intussusceptum may strangulate and infarct. Abdominal examination may reveal a mass and occasionally the apex of the intussusception may protrude from the anus or be felt on rectal examination.

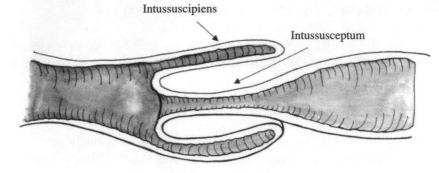

Figure 7.1. Intussusception.

In children most intussusceptions are thought to be caused by peristalsis acting on a hypertophied Peyer's patch Meckel's diverticulum is another possible cause. Sometimes the intussusception can be reduced by a barium enema (so-called hydrostatic reducton), and if this is unsuccessful, surgical correction is required. If possible the intussusception is simply reduced and recurrence is then uncommon. If it cannot be reduced or if it is nonviable, then the affected segment needs to be resected.

If intussusception occurs in an adult (which is rare), then a tumour (benign or malignant) acting as the apex of the intussusception should be considered.

ACUTE APPENDICITIS

Acute appendicitis is the commonest emergency surgical presentation requiring operation. Most cases are thought to be caused by obstruction of the appendix with subsequent infection behind the obstruction. This concept of an obstructed system getting infected is also relevant to conditions such as cholangitis (infection of an obstructed biliary tree) and pylonephritis (infection of an obstructed renal tract). In appendicitis the most common cause of obstruction of the appendix is either from a faecolith (a piece of faeces within the appendix) or hypertrophy of lymphoid tissue within the wall of the appendix, presumably in response to an otherwise minor viral infection. Rare causes of obstruction of the appendix and therefore appendicitis include carcinoma of the caecum and carcinoid tumour.

To understand the way in which appendicitis presents clinically, one should realise that in its early stages the inflammation of the appendix is confined to the wall of the appendix itself and is therefore felt as a poorly localised visceral pain in the central abdominal. Because the essential feature is of an obstructed appendix, the pain will usually be colicky due to peristalsis in the appendicular muscle. As the inflammatory process progresses the surrounding tissues and parietal peritoneum become inflamed and the pain is then felt locally in the right iliac fossa and is constant and typical of a localised peritonitis, worse on movement, etc. The typical patient will therefore present with an initial central colicky abdominal pain, which after a few hours progresses into a constant right iliac fossa pain (the pain moves; it does not radiate). By this time the patient will usually have a mild fever, be anorexic and may have nausea and vomiting. On examination there will be localised right iliac fossa tenderness and guarding with rebound tenderness or percussion tenderness. The diagnosis is essentially a clinical one and in straightforward cases no investigations at all are required.

The treatment of acute appendicitis is appendicectomy. It would be very reasonable of an examiner to ask simple questions about the operation, as it is the most common one performed as an emergency. For that reason the basic steps of an appendicectomy will be outlined.

First of all, an incision is made in the right iliac fossa. Conventionally this would be centred over McBurney's point, which is two thirds the way along a line drawn from the umbilicus to the anterior superior iliac spine. In practice many surgeons make a slightly lower incision, which is cosmetically more acceptable. However, McBurney's point is often asked about in examinations because it marks the usual site of the base of the appendix. An incision is then made down through skin and subcutaneous tissues until the muscle layers are reached. The external oblique, internal oblique and transverse abdominus muscles are then opened. This is done by a muscle-splitting incision along the lines of the fibres with no fibres actually being cut. The final layer is the peritoneum, which is opened so that the abdominal cavity can be entered. The appendix and caecum are then identified and pulled up through the incision. There seems to be a misconception among many medical students that the retrocaecal appendix is unusual. In fact this is the commonest site of the appendix. After delivery of the appendix the blood vessels and mesentery of the appendix are divided and the appendix is ligated and removed at its base. Many surgeons then bury the stump of the appendix with a purse-string suture around the caecum. The caecum is then returned to the abdomen. Any fluid or pus is carefully sucked and swabbed out. If there is severe contamination a drain may be left. The layers of the abdominal muscles are then closed using an absorbable suture. The operation should be covered with prophylactic antibiotics, usually Metronidazole, given intravenously at induction of the anaesthetic.

Another misconception that many students (and indeed doctors) have relates to the presence of tenderness on rectal examination. Only 7% of appendixes lie in a pelvic position and most of these do not reach far enough into the pelvis to be in any way near to an examining finger. Therefore, when patients have rectal tenderness in association with acute appendicitis, it is not because of the adjacent position of the inflamed appendix; it is in fact because inflammatory fluids and perhaps pus have tracted down from the area of the appendix in the right iliac fossa to the most dependent portion of the abdominal cavity, the pouch of Douglas.

Occasionally, acute appendicitis may present after it has been fully walled off by the omentum and small bowel. At this stage (usually greater than 72 h after the onset of symptoms) a mass is usually present on palpation. This may either resolve on antibiotics or develop into an abscess. Some surgeons may advocate an "interval" appendicectomy at

Causes of a Right Iliac Fossa Mass

1. Appendix mass
2. Gynaecological mass (e.g. ovarian cyst)
3. Caecal cancer
4. Soft tissue tumour, e.g. sarcoma
5. Lymph node mass
6. TB
7. Actinomycosis
8. Transplant kidney
9. Iliac aneurysm

about three months (Ochsner–Sherren regimen) whilst others would perform an appendicectomy during the initial admission.

MESENTERIC ADENITIS

Mesenteric adenitis is the main differential diagnosis for acute appendicitis. It is a condition where enlargement of the mesenteric lymph nodes occurs, causing pain and a temperature, as well as local tenderness. It is mostly seen in children and adolescents and is often associated with a viral or upper respiratory tract infection. Headache and photophobia are more common than acute appendicitis. The temperature is often higher than in acute appendicitis and the tenderness and pain may not be as focal. Investigation shows a lymphocytosis rather than a raised neutrophil count. No specific treatment other than paracetamol is usually required.

SMALL BOWEL OBSTRUCTION

The commonest cause of small bowel obstruction in the western world is adhesions, secondary to previous surgery, and the second-commonest cause is hernias. Other causes can be classified as in the following table.

Causes of Intestinal Obstruction

In the Lumen
- Impacted faeces or food bolus obstruction
- Swallowed foreign body
- Large polyps
- Intussusception

In the Wall
- Tumours
- Infarction
- Crohn's disease
- Benign stricture

Outside the Wall
- Adhesions
- Strangulated hernia
- Volvulus
- Extrinsic compression

The precise symptoms and presentation depend on the site of the obstruction, but the four cardinal features are:

1. Pain
2. Abdominal distension
3. Vomiting
4. Absolute constipation

The pain is usually colicky in nature, i.e. intermittent spasms of pain due to peristalsis which wear off after a few seconds, only to return a few minutes later. The pain is often severe and makes the patient double up whilst it is present. Pain due to small bowel obstruction is usually found in the central abdomen. Distension is variable and depends on the level of the obstruction, with more distal obstruction causing greater degrees of distension, as one might expect. Likewise, vomiting occurs early with high intestinal obstruction and late with low intestinal obstruction. Absolute constipation means that the patient is passing neither flatus nor faeces. In a high obstruction absolute constipation may not be present.

Abdominal examination may reveal distension and runs of hyperactive bowel sounds. Focal tenderness implies that strangulation might be occurring. "Strangulation" refers to compromise of part of the intestinal blood supply due to twisting or kinking of its mesentery. It may also be suggested by findings of a temperature or raised white count and obviously in later stages will progress to gangrene and perforation of the bowel with signs of generalised peritonitis. A plain abdominal X-ray may be helpful in confirming the diagnosis of small bowel obstruction. The typical appearance would be of distended small bowel loops (remember that the small bowel usually has a diameter of less than 4 cm on a plain X-ray and is characterised by its central position within the abdomen and valvulae conniventes which go all the way across the bowel lumen).

Treatment of Small Bowel Obstruction

The patient should be carefully assessed and on abdominal examination particular attention should be paid to the presence of previous abdominal scars or the presence of hernias. The groin should be very carefully examined, as a small femoral hernia can be easily missed unless specifically looked for. If a hernia is found in a patient who is obstructed, then immediate surgery is required to repair the hernia and release the obstruction, as it is likely that the bowel is strangulated within the hernia. At operation the bowel should be carefully inspected, and if it is thought to be nonviable a resection of that section of the bowel may be required. If the obstruction is thought to be due to adhesions and if there are no suggestions that strangulation has already occurred, then a period of conservative management may be appropriate. This usually consists of placing the patient "nil by mouth", passing a nasogastric tube which should be left on free drainage with two-hourly aspiration in an attempt to decompress the bowel, and giving intravenous fluids to avoid dehydration ("drip and suck"). The patient should then be carefully monitored and the resolution of the obstruction would be marked by a lessening of pain, a decrease in the NGT aspirate volumes, the passage of flatus and the resolution of signs on a repeat X-ray. Should the patient not settle within 24 h or should signs of strangulation develop, then surgery would be indicated. Surgery for adhesions normally consists of a laparotomy at which the adhesions are divided.

The term "subacute bowel obstruction" is sometimes used to describe the condition where only one or two of the four cardinal signs are present. However, this term is really meaningless and obstruction should be classified as complete or partial. There is one other term used, which is "pseudo-obstruction". This means the patient is obstructed but no mechanical cause can be found and it may be due to many factors, such as electrolyte abnormalities.

LARGE BOWEL OBSTRUCTION

The commonest causes of acute large bowel obstruction are carcinoma of the colon, diverticulitis and volvulus of the sigmoid or caecum. Unlike small bowel obstruction, adhesions and hernias are rarer causes. Like small bowel obstruction, large bowel obstruction gives rise to distension, colicky abdominal pain, vomiting and constipation; although vomiting may take longer to onset. In 20% of people the ileocaecal valve is competent and decompression of the large bowel back into the small bowel cannot occur. This is a dangerous situation, as pressure can rapidly build up in the colon, leading to a perforation, which is the major complication in large bowel obstruction. Perforation usually occurs in the caecum, as this is the thinnest-walled and most distensible part of the colon. Investigations would be blood tests (FBC, U & E, amylase and group and save) and X-rays. Sigmoidoscopy may show the site of the lesion and an emergency contrast enema may be helpful in differentiating true from pseudo-obstruction. Management is intravenous resuscitation and passage of a nasogastric tube. Immediate laparotomy is indicated if signs of peritonitis are present (indicating perforation has occurred) or if the caecum is greater than 10 cm in diameter or very tender, indicating imminent perforation.

INFLAMMATORY BOWEL DISEASE

Inflammatory bowel disease is a term which includes both ulcerative colitis and Crohn's disease.

Crohn's Disease

Crohn's disease is a chronic relapsing, transmural granulomatous disorder (i.e. on histology the whole thickness of the bowel is affected and granulomas are seen) of unknown aetiology. It can occur anywhere in the gastrointestinal tract, from mouth to anus, but is commonest in the terminal ileum (hence its old name, "terminal ileitis"). It can affect the colon, where occasionally it may be difficult to differentiate from ulcerative colitis. It will often affect separate areas of bowel with normal bowel in between (so-called "skip" lesions). It tends to produce healing by fibrosis resulting in strictures and has a tendency to form fistulae to other structures, such as adjacent loops of bowel, the bladder, the vagina and the skin surface.

The way in which Crohn's disease first presents varies with its site and extent. The commonest presentation will be with a change in the bowel habit, usually diarrhoea, central abdominal colicky pains or pains in the right iliac fossa, fever, anorexia, weight loss and general malaise. On examination there may be tenderness or a mass in the abdomen, most often in the right iliac fossa. Often, however, there are no abnormal physical signs. Investigation consists of the exclusion of other possible diagnoses, including carcinoma. Blood tests may be helpful and show elevated acute phase proteins, especially C reactive protein. The mainstay of diagnosis, however, involves contrast studies (barium follow-through examination of the small bowel or barium enema for the colon) and endoscopic studies with biopsy (e.g. colonoscopy).

Most cases of Crohn's disease are initially managed medically by gastroenterologists, although about 65% will at some time require surgery. Drugs such as Mesalazine and steroids may be used. Severe cases where there is stricture formation, fistualization or an inflammatory mass that is not resolving, may need surgical intervention.

The surgery for Crohn's disease depends on which part of the bowel is affected and the treatment can be divided into surgery for small and large bowel disease.

If the small bowel is predominantly involved, the main aims of surgery will be to perform stricturoplasties or resect the very diseased bowel locally but to minimise resection as much as possible. The reason for this is that occasional patients may require repeated surgery and end up with short gut syndrome if too much bowel is resected (the patients' main concern is liquid stools, although they also have all the vitamin and nutritional deficiencies). In large bowel disease the operation usually performed is panproctocolectomy with ileostomy (removal of the whole large bowel and anus). This is because smaller, more limited resections of the large bowel in Crohn's are associated with high relapse rates requiring further surgery.

Detailed questions about Crohn's disease are most likely to come from gastroenterologists in medical exams. However, you should obviously know about the associated complications outside the abdomen, including the high incidence of perianal disease such as abscesses and perianal fistulae, the skin changes of erythema nodosum and pyoderma gangraenosum, the associated arthritis and occular problems, etc.

Ulcerative Colitis

Unlike Crohn's disease, ulcerative colitis (UC) affects only the colon, and whilst Crohn's disease affects the full thickness of the bowel wall, ulcerative colitis affects only the mucosa. Another difference from Crohn's disease is that UC usually affects the rectum and as the disease gets more extensive it spreads proximally in a continual pattern (i.e. skip lesions should make one consider Crohn's disease). Like Crohn's disease, UC is a chronic and relapsing condition. The normal mode of presentation will be of blood-stained diarrhoea and abdominal pain, which is often eased by defaecation (NB: UC tends to be bloody diarrhoea whereas Crohn's tends to be painful diarrhoea). In most cases there are no abnormal physical signs. In more severe cases nausea, vomiting and distension may occur in association with pyrexia, and this should make one suspect the development of toxic megacolon.

In nonacute cases investigation consists of the elimination of other pathologies, and confirmation is usually made by biopsy on sigmoidoscopy or colonoscopy. It can sometimes be difficult for the histologist to differentiate Crohn's from UC, and he then terms the condition as "indeterminate" or nonspecific inflammatory bowel disease. The other major difference between Crohn's disease and UC is that while the former appears to have only a small premalignant potential, the latter is most definitely premalignant. The figure usually quoted is that for ulcerative colitis involving most of the colon there is a 10% risk of developing a carcinoma for every ten years that the disease exists. Because of this people with UC are advised to have regular routine screening colonoscopies with biopsies every two to three years. The particular feature looked for on the biopsy is the development of dysplasia, and if it is severe, consideration should be given to the possibility of an elective total colectomy to reduce the risk of cancer formation. The operation will normally be a panproctocdectomy, which means that the whole of the colon, rectum and anus will be removed so that no colonic mucosa will be left. After this the patient either is left with a terminal ileostomy or can have a new pelvic reservoir constructed ("a pouch"), which is made by joining several loops of small bowel together and sewing that directly down to the anal sphincters. A pouch operation would nowadays normally be offered to any young person requiring a total colectomy for UC. Such an operation cannot be offered to patients with Crohn's colitis, because Crohn's disease often recurs in the small bowel used to construct the reservoir and the results of the operation are therefore poor.

The majority of UC patients (> 85%) can be managed medcially (antidiarrhoeals, steroids, Mesalazine, etc.), unlike Crohn's disease, in which about 65% will require surgery at some point. The principal acute complication of UC which you need to know about and which might require surgical intervention is toxic megacolon. This is diagnosed on a plain X-ray and is defined as dilatation of the transverse colon above 6 cm. The patient will normally be quite unwell with UC and will present with severe blood-stained diarrhoea and systemic signs such as fever, dehydration and tachycardia. There is usually abdominal tenderness and the white cell count may be raised. Initial attempts will usually be made to treat the patient conservatively with intravenous fluids and high dose intravenous steroids. Repeated abdominal X-rays should be taken to watch the size of the colon (usually the transverse colon), and if it appears to be getting bigger despite appropriate medical treatment an operation is indicated before it perforates. Also, if a perforation is suspected or if the patient fails to settle within 24–48 h of medical treatment, then surgery will be indicated.

In this situation the usual surgical procedure is a total colectomy, an ileostomy, and the rectal stump is usually also brought out to the skin so that it can be inspected (this is called a mucous fistula). Subsequently, when the acute problem has settled, the patient could be offered an ileal reservoir or completion colectomy (i.e. removal of the rest of the rectum and anus, leaving them with a permanant ileostomy) according to discussions between the surgeon and patient.

It is not uncommon to get shown a barium enema during your viva, and the commonest diagnoses are ulcerative colitis or an apple core stricture indicating malignancy. You may also get shown a barium meal with follow-through which looks at the small bowel (you see some contrast in the stomach and hence you can tell it is a follow-through), and this may show the strictures of Crohn's disease.

COLON CANCER

Colon cancer is the commonest gastrointestinal cancer and questions are therefore common in surgical finals. Patients who have had previous operations for colon cancer are often brought up as long cases.

The way in which colon cancer presents depends partly on its position within the colon. Tumours on the right side of the colon are more likely to present later with a mass or anaemia, since the faeces are still liquid in this region and thus are less likely to produce an obstruction to the flow. In contradistinction, tumours on the left side of the colon are more likely to present early with obstruction and a change in the bowel habit.

Tumours in the rectum may give rise to tenesmus, which is a symptom where the patient feels as though there are some faeces which they need to pass even after they have just emptied their bowels. This symptom is actually a reflection of the mass present within the rectum.

Examination may be entirely normal. Rectal examination is mandatory, as you may be able to feel a low rectal tumour. Flexible sigmoidoscopy should also be performed, which will allow visualisation (and biopsy) of tumours in the last 15 cm or so of the intestinal tract (which may be missed on barium enema).

Investigations — simple blood tests (FBC, U & E, LFT's) and CEA (carcino-embryonic antigen — a marker for bowel cancer) — should be measured. Further investigation is usually with barium enema (apple core lesion) or colonoscopy, where a stricture or mass will be found. Colonoscopy allows biopsies to be taken. Ultrasound or CT may be indicated to stage and screen for liver metastases.

A common question relates to the staging of colon cancer. The classical way of staging such tumours is the Dukes staging. Initially Sir Cuthbert Dukes (a pathologist at St Mark's Hospital, London) described three stages: Type A, where the tumour is confined to the bowel wall (this has a 90% five-year survival rate); Type B, where the tumour has invaded through the bowel wall into surrounding tissue but the lymph nodes are clear (this has a 60% five-year survival rate); Type C, where the lymph nodes are involved, and this stage is usually divided into C1 and C2. C1 is where lymph nodes are involved only up to the resection margins. C2 is where the highest lymph node in the surgical specimen is involved (implying further spread). Overall, stage C has a five-year survival of about 30%. Although not originally described by Dukes, the further stage D is now usually mentioned where there is distant spread, and this has a 5–10% five-year survival rate. The treatment of colon cancer is surgery and resection of the tumour. Preoperatively patients should have bowel preparation. Tumours of the right colon usually undergo right hemicolectomy, the transverse colon a transverse colectomy, and the descending colon tumours undergo left hemicolectomy. When resecting bowel cancers attention is paid to the blood supply to the segment involved. There must be a good blood supply to the two cut ends and, therefore, the surgeon removes the entire part of the bowel supplied by the same blood vessels as those supplying the tumour (and hence are ligated when the tumour is resected). Thus a tumour of the caecum (supplied by the right colic artery) means a right hemicolectomy.

Tumours of the rectum are treated by anterior resection (this is where the rectal tumour is removed and the colon above the tumour is anastomosed to the remaining rectal stump). Usually a primary anastomosis is performed using either sutures or a staple gun. If the immediate strength of the anastomosis is in doubt, then a proximal temporary stoma (usually an ileostomy or a transverse colostomy) may be constructed and closed a few weeks later. This is in order to divert the faeces away from the healing anastomosis.

If the tumour is very low down and excision cannot be performed without damaging the anal sphincters, then an abdominoperineal (AP) resection (i.e. excision of the rectum and anus leaving the patient with a permanent colostomy) is required. This is a much more extensive operation and leaves the patient with two wounds (the perineal and the laparotomy) and a colostomy.

In terms of the latest developments in the understanding of rectal cancer, it is now thought that the presence of radial spread (in an outward direction from the bowel into the surrounding mesentry) is an important prognostic indicator and therefore many surgeons nowadays perform a careful total mesorectal excision (removing the mesentery of the bowel) during an anterior resection in order to reduce the incidence of local recurrence.

The role of adjuvant therapy in colorectal cancer is still unclear. Many studies have been published and many more are still underway. At present it appears that systemic chemotherapy with 5-Fluorouracil and levamisole leads to increased survival and decreased recurrence in patients with Dukes C cancers. The role of chemotherapy in Dukes B cancers is less clear.

Radiotherapy is of no value in colon cancer (as the tumour is too mobile and not particularly radiosensitive) but may have a role in some rectal tumours.

Stomas and Types of Colonic Resectons

Questions on these are common. The following is a simple guide.

A stoma in the right lower quadrant is usually an ileostomy. Because small bowel content is irritant to the skin, ileostomies are usually constructed with a spout and they stand clear of the skin by a few centimetres. They may be either an end ileostomy in someone who has had a total colectomy or a loop ileostomy where the bowel has been temporarily "defunctioned". This latter type is usually performed after a difficult colonic resection to give the anastomosis time to heal before restoring intestinal continuity. Obviously, the end ileostomy will have only one opening whilst the loop ileostomy will have two. However, students will not usually be expected to remove ileostomy bags to confirm this in exams. There can be large fluid losses from an ileostomy and it is important to regularly measure these losses and replace them accordingly via the drip to prevent dehydration.

A stoma in the right upper quadrant is usually a defunctioning transverse colostomy. Like the defunctioning ileostomy, it will have two lumens, but will not usually have a spout and is therefore flush with the skin surface. Again it will usually be a temporary stoma to cover an anastomosis or occasionally a severe attack of diverticulitis with obstruction.

Stomas are not usually constructed in the left upper quadrant; however, if there is one it is probably one of the types found in the left lower quadrant, which for technical reasons has been sited higher than usual.

Left lower quadrant stomas may be either end colostomies, loop colostomies or double-barrelled colostomies. An end colostomy is produced after resection of the rectum or sigmoid colon. There is an operation called Hartman's procedure, in which part of the rectum is resected and the rectal stump is left inside the pelvis and closed with sutures, while a temporary end colostomy is brought out in the left lower quadrant. This is most often performed for perforated diverticulitis, where the affected portion of bowel is resected but the contamination makes it unsafe to join the ends back together immediately. A permanent end colostomy is produced after complete excision of the anus and rectum

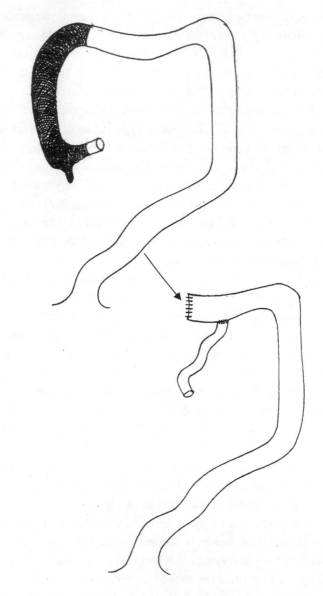

Figure 7.2(a). Colonic resections. Right hemicolectomy.

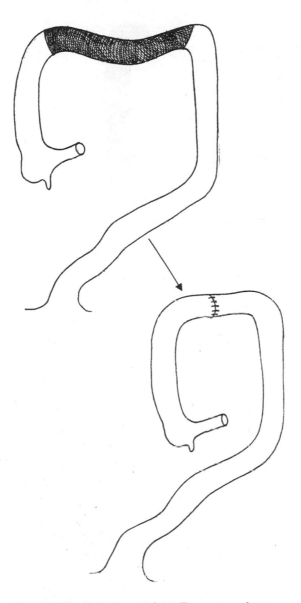

Figure 7.2(b). Colonic resections. Transverse colectomy.

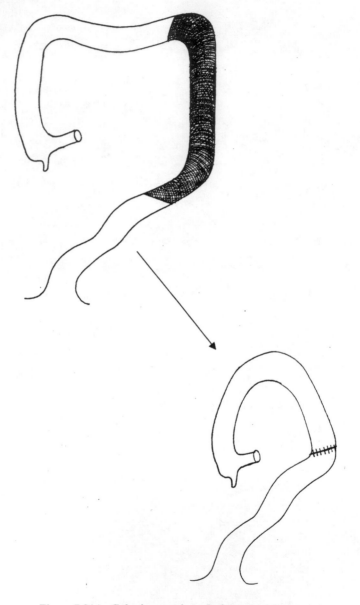

Figure 7.2(c). Colonic resections. Left hemicolectomy.

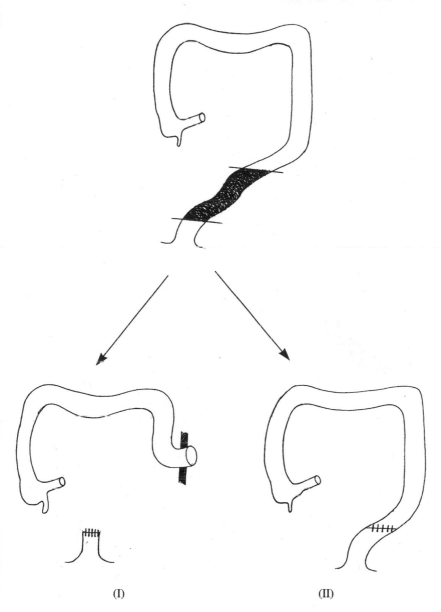

(I)   (II)

Figure 7.2(d). Colonic resections. Surgery for disease of the sigmoid colon or rectum —
(I) Hartman's, (II) sigmoid colectomy. The decision about which operation is performed
depends on several factors, including the disease process, the skill of the surgeon and
the general health of the patient.

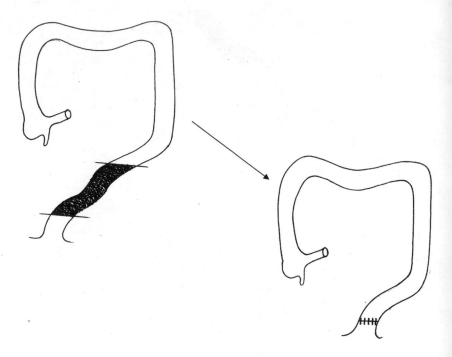

Figure 7.2(e). Colonic resections. Anterior resection.

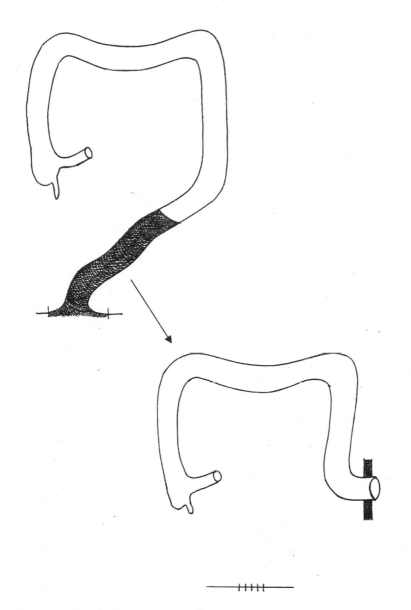

Figure 7.2(f). Colonic resections. Abdominoperineal resection (note that there are two wounds — the laparotomy and the perineal wound — and a stoma).

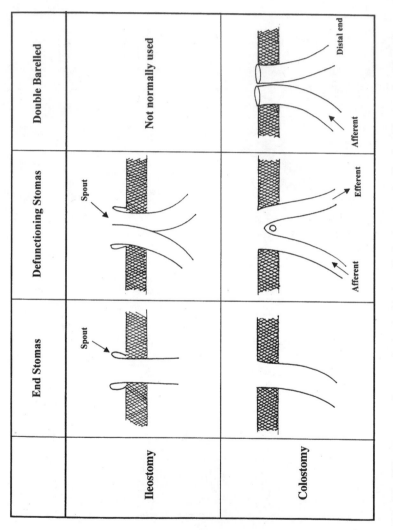

Figure 7.3. The different types of stomas. In the double-barrelled colostomy the distal end is sometimes known as a mucous fistula. This allows it to be inspected and reversal, if necessary, is easier.

(an abdominoperineal excision) for a very low rectal cancer. If after a resection it is thought unsafe to join the bowel ends together, but the distal end is long enough, then both ends may be brought out together to the surface. This is called a double-barrelled colostomy. If the bowel is long enough, it is preferred to a Hartmann's, because reversal does not require a full relaparotomy. Loop colostomy is when the apex of the sigmoid is brought out as a stoma without a resection having been performed. This is occasionally done for an inoperable carcinoma of the rectum that is likely to obstruct.

Screening for Colorectal Cancer

Colonoscopy is the ideal test but is expensive. The haemoccult test, which looks for faecal occult blood, is one of the better and cheaper tests. However, it has a relatively low sensitivity and gives a high false positive rate; even so studies that are under way, looking at the haemoccult test, show early indications of a decreased mortality in the screened groups.

There are no clear guides as to who should be screened for polyps or colorectal cancer. However, the following should be screened:

(1) Those with familial adenomatous polyposis (who usually have a colectomy early).
(2) Strong family history (more than two close relatives).
(3) Anyone with a personal history of polyps or colorectal cancer.
(4) Patients with ulcerative colitis for more than 10 years, Peutz–Jeghers, juvenile polyposis, etc.

Carcinoembryonic antigen (CEA) is a serological marker for colorectal cancer. However, it is not usually elevated in early disease (less than 5% of Dukes A cancers have a raised CEA) and it also has low specificity, being raised in many other conditions (such as other inflammatory conditions of the GI tract, smoking or renal impairment). Therefore, it has little value in any screening programme. It is, however, used in the follow-up of patients with colorectal cancer. The level of

CEA should fall to normal limits within weeks of the operation to remove the cancer. At the follow-up clinics a rise in CEA can be used to diagnose recurrence of the tumour, often before it is clinically apparent.

Colonic Polyps

A polyp is defined as "a lesion which projects into the lumen of the bowel". The relevance in the colon is mainly because of the tendency of some types of polyps to become malignant. The general term "polyp", however, is purely a morphological term and in no way defines the actual diagnosis for which histology would usually be required (most often obtained by biopsy at sigmoidoscopy or colonoscopy). It is helpful to consider polyps under their different pathological headings:

(1) *Adenomatous Polyps*

Adenomatous polyps are important because of their tendency to lead to colorectal cancer. Most authorities believe that the majority of adenocarcinomas of the colon develop from pre-existing adenomatous polyps. Evidence for this belief includes the fact that early stages of malignancy (severe dysplasia and carcinoma *in situ*) may sometimes be found in polyps and that patients with familial adenomatous polyposis die of cancer at a young age unless they have a prophylactic colectomy. In addition, carcinogens which produce adenomas experimentally also lead to cancer formation, and studies in which patients were followed up after previous colorectal cancer in which polyps were prophylactically removed at colonoscopy, appeared to have a reduced incidence of subsequent new cancer development. The likelihood of an adenomatous polyp becoming malignant seemed to relate to its size. It appears to be rare for adenomas under 1 cm in size but occurs with increasing likelihood as the polyp gets bigger. Adenomatous polyps of the colon are usually subclassified into the better-differentiated tubular adenomas (75%), which are often on a stalk, and the less-differentiated villous adenomas (10%), which are often sessile (i.e. flat). Sometimes a polyp is described as tubulovillous

(15%) when it has an appearance somewhere between these two extremes.

Adenomas can be sporadic or familial. The familial adenomas occur in conditions such as familial multiple polyposis coli and gardener's syndrome, and they have a high if not inevitable chance of developing into cancer.

Familial multiple polyposis coli is an autosomal dominant condition with multiple neoplastic colonic polyps beginning in the second to third decade, and patients usually have a prophylactic colectomy in their early twenties.

Gardeners' syndrome is an autosomal dominant condition with multiple colonic adenomas in association with bony osteomas and epidermoid cysts.

Other than being premalignant, adenomatous polyps may present with the following:

- Bleeding which may be either frank blood or microscopic bleeding (present with anaemia).
- Polyps rarely present with change in the bowel habit, but a large benign polyp in the rectum can produce the symptoms of tenesmus (i.e. a sensation of incomplete evacuation due to the presence of a mass within the rectum).
- Some polyps may also secrete a large amount of mucus and the patient may complain of passing slime or jelly.
- Rarely, a polyp will prolapse through the anus or act as the apex for an intussusception.

Polyps may be diagnosed on imaging the colon with a barium enema, but if suspected the best investigation is usually a colonoscopy which gives the additional advantage of providing the opportunity for biopsy or complete removal of the polyp. Key points on histology, other than the diagnosis of an adenomatous polyp, will be whether or not there is any evidence of dysplasia of the cells on the surface of the polyp. Most histologists would classify this as mild, moderate or severe, with severe dysplasia being strongly suggestive that the lesion was premalignant.

(2) *Hamartomatous Polyps*

A hamartoma (a lesion where there is an overgrowth of one or more of the cell types which are normal constituents of the organ from which they arise) is an unusual lesion defined as an abnormality of development. With regard to colonic polyps, there are two conditions in which hamartomatous polyps are normally described:

- *Juvenile polyps.* These have a low malignant potential. They may present with bleeding or intussusception and sometimes slough off spontaneously and actually present with material passed in the motion and noticed by the patient or parents. Usually it is possible to deal with them colonoscopically.
- *Peutz–Jeghers syndrome.* This is a rare autosomal dominant condition where multiple hamartomatous polyps appear throughout the entire gastrointestinal tract and the affected individuals also have pigmentation of the skin around the lips and gums. Again the malignant potential of these polyps is small, although overall the patient is at a greater risk of developing carcinoma (both GI and non-GI tract).

(3) *Polyps Due to Protrusions of Mesenchymal Tissue*

Conditions such as lipomas (benign tumours of fat), leiomyomas (benign tumours of smooth muscle), neurofibromas (benign tumours arising from nerve tissue) and haemangiomas (benign tumours of blood vessel origin) can all occur in the wall of the colon, and if they then form a lump which protrudes into the lesion they are by definition polyps. These are all rather rare in clinical practice and their main importance is that they may mimic the presentation of a carcinoma.

(4) *Metaplastic Polyps*

These are sometimes also call hyperplastic polyps. They are usually small, often multiple and slightly raised above the surrounding normal mucosa. They have a distinctive histological appearance and have no malignant potential whatsoever. Because of their small size they cause no symptoms and their only relevance is in distinguishing them from adenomatous polyps. They are often seen in inflammatory bowel disease or lymphoid hyperplasia (such as at the appendix). If they are found incidentally at appendicectomy, then usually no other treatment is required.

(5) *Inflammatory Polyps*

Examples are those found in inflammatory conditions of the bowel, such as pseudopolyps in ulcerative colitis.

Diverticular Disease

Diverticulae are defined as out-pouchings from a tubular structure (the opposite of polyps).

Chronic diverticulac occur where the colonic mucosa bulges out at the weakest point where blood vessels enter the colonic muscle. They tend to appear in middle and old age and are much more common in western countries, where it is thought that they may be caused by lack of fibre in the diet leading to muscle spasm and hence increased intraluminal pressure and bulging-out of the mucosa. They are usually found on the left side of the colon, although they can occasionally involve all of the colon around as far as the caecum. They are extremely common, being found in the majority of elderly patients, especially if there is a history of constipation. Many are asymptomatic, but diverticular disease can be responsible for a number of clinical problems:

(1) Chronic symptoms of *gripey abdominal pains*, diarrhoea and passage of pellety stools are often ascribed to diverticular disease. Normal treatment is usually with antispasmodics and a high fibre diet.
(2) *Acute diverticulitis.* This is a condition where a diverticulum becomes inflamed, usually because of the presence of inspissated faeces within it. In many ways it is similar to the process involved in acute appendicitis, and indeed diverticulitis is sometimes called "left-sided appendicitis". The typical presentation would be an elderly patient, perhaps with a previous history of problems with constipation etc., who presents with pain and tenderness in the left

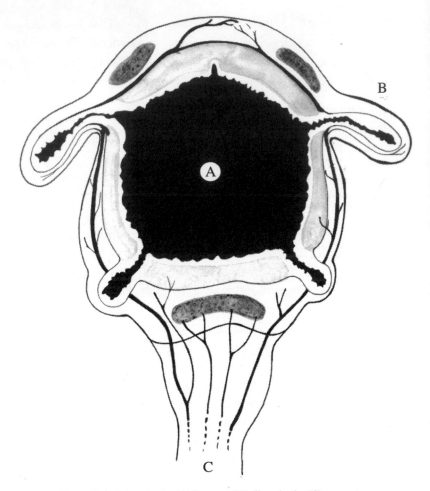

Figure 7.4. Diverticula. (A) Lumen, (B) diverticula, (C) mesentry.

iliac fossa, a fever, local signs of peritonitis and a raised white cell count. The majority of cases of acute diverticulitis can be treated successfully with conservative management consisting of resting the bowel, intravenous fluids and antibiotics. If they do not settle or their symptoms worsen, then they may require surgical intervention.

(3) *Perforated diverticulitis.* Some patients may present with a more sudden onset of pain, perhaps preceded by signs and symptoms

suggestive of acute diverticulitis, and have more generalised signs of peritonitis on examination. In addition they may be shocked or have free gas on an erect chest X-ray, indicating a perforation. These patients will usually require laparotomy for confirmation of the diagnosis, washing out of contamination from the abdominal cavity and usually resection of the sigmoid colon, often as a Hartmann's procedure where the affected sigmoid colon is resected, the lower end (the rectal stump) is oversewn and left within the pelvis, and the proximal end is brought out usually as a temporary left iliac fossa colostomy (which can be reversed after a few months). See Figure 7.2.

(4) *Diverticular abscess.* Sometimes a perforated diverticulum, rather than leading to free peritonitis, is walled off by surrounding anatomical structures such as bowel loops and leads to a local abscess formation. If a mass is felt on examination and this diagnosis is suspected, then the investigation of choice is probably a CT. Treatment is as for acute diverticulitis initially (the outline of the mass can be marked on the skin for regular reassessment), and if the patient fails to respond then drainage, either surgical or radiological, is needed. Sometimes the patient requires a resection and Hartmann's procedure as above.

(5) *Haemorrhage.* This is usually sudden and painless, and there can be bright or dark red blood. It usually stops spontaneously, although if it persists angiography and surgery may be required to remove the affected part of the bowel.

(6) *Stricture of the colon.* After the resolution of acute diverticulitis the colon may sometimes heal with a fibrous stricture formation. If severe this may require resection. Usually, when a resection is performed in the absence of acute inflammation or an abscess, it is possible to join the ends of the bowel together again immediately, with either sutures or staples, i.e. performing a "primary anastomosis". Other causes of a colonic stricture include a carcinoma, ulcerative colitis or Crohn's disease, ischaemic colitis, postradiotherapy changes or surgery — at the site of an anastomosis.

Lower Gastrointestinal Bleeding

This is caused by a number of possible conditions. It is, like upper gastrointestinal bleeding, a common question in finals. The mainstay of investigation is colonoscopy and patients only occasionally require emergency surgery. Remember, if answering a question, to deal initially with rapid assessment and treatment of the shocked patient.

The causes of a lower GI bleed are:

- Haemorrhoids
- Carcinoma
- Diverticular disease
- Angiodysplasia
- Infective colitis
- Polyps
- Fistula
- Ulcerative colitis

The age of the patient is important — for example, haemorrhoids, cancer, diverticular diease and angiodysplasia are the most common in elderly patients, whereas infective colitis and ulcerative colitis are more common in young people.

In the history note the frequency and amount of bleeding, the colour (bright red blood is suggestive of lower GI bleeding, whereas dark red blood could be both upper or lower GI bleeding), whether the bleeding was associated with the passage of faeces and if so whether it was mixed in, whether there was any mucus or slime and whether there was any abdominal pain (suggestive of inflammatory disease).

Examination should always include a proctoscopy (and if possible a rigid sigmoidoscopy) to look for a local cause of bleeding (e.g. haemorrhoids). Resuscitation is the same as that for an upper GI bleed, although many cases stop bleeding spontaneously. If this is the case and there was a significant bleed, then the patient is admitted for a barium enema or colonoscopy to find the source of bleeding. If the bleed was small and stops spontaneously, then the patient may be able to be investigated as an out-patient. Very occasionally the bleeding continues and is rapid, requiring an urgent angiogram to find the source of the bleeding. If a region of the bowel is shown to have abnormal blood vessels (i.e. angiodysplasia), then surgery to remove the affected area may be required (occasionally the bleeding vessel can be stopped by embolizing the vessel radiologically). The operation required will depend on where the cause of the bleeding is.

In some cases it is impossible to tell from the history whether the bleed was from the upper or the lower GI tract, and in these cases the patient needs a gastroscopy initially to rule out an upper GI lesion.

8

RECTUM AND ANUS

HAEMORRHOIDS

There is much debate in surgical circles about the true nature of haemorrhoids. Unfortunately this sometimes manifests itself in finals by questions such as "What exactly are haemorrhoids?". They are probably a vascular cushion, covered in a layer of mucosa and containing a branch of the superior rectal artery and a tributary of the superior rectal vein. The key point that the examiners will want you to make is that haemorrhoids are not simply dilated veins (when they bleed the blood is bright red). Haemorrhoids occur at the point where the superior rectal branches enter the muscle. Conventionally their position is described in relation to the anus imagined as a clock face visualized with the patient in the lithotomy position (i.e. on his back with his legs up in stirrups). In this position the penis or vagina is anterior at 12 o'clock and the scrotum posterior at 6 o'clock. There are usually three haemorrhoids, at 3, 7 and 11 o'clock.

Haemorrhoids are classified as follows:

1st degree — they do not prolapse from the anus.
2nd degree — they prolapse on defaecaton or straining but return spontaneously.
3rd degree — they prolapse and remain prolapsed unless manually repositioned.

Haemorrhoids may be asymptomatic, although if they do cause symptoms this is usually bleeding or minor pain and itching. They are usually not severely painful unless they are prolapsed and thrombosed. Bleeding from haemorrhoids is usually bright red and either on the outside of the motion or on the toilet paper. There is usually no change in the fundamental bowel habit and no other gastrointestinal symptoms or signs. Haemorrhoids can be treated by injection (with 5% phenol in almond oil); this works by shrinking the haemorrhoid through causing scar formation, by rubber band ligation or by coagulation with infrared devices. These procedures are usually performed in the out-patient department. If these methods fail, then it may be necessary to formally excise the haemorrhoids ("haemorrhoidectomy"), as a day case or an in-patient procedure.

Fissure *in Ano*

A fissure *in ano* usually starts with a tear in the anal canal caused by trauma or the passage of a constipated stool. In some cases this fails to heal and the inflammation it produces causes spasm in the sphincter muscle so that further trauma occurs when motions are passed and it eventually becomes a chronic fissure. Examination it often painful and it may be possible to see an external hypertrophic skin tag "sentinel pile", which is indurated at the base where the fissure lies.

The initial treatment for a fissure is conservative, with advice to avoid straining on the toilet (and the use of bulk laxatives) and the topical application of local anaesthetic gels. If these methods fail, then surgery may be needed. In the past the surgical treatment was manual dilatation of the anus under a general anaesthetic, but this was associated with high rates of long term incontinence. Nowadays, chronic fissure is usually treated by the operation of lateral subcutaneous sphincterotomy, in which the external sphincter is partially divided through a small laterally placed stab incision. NB: The latest research is into the use of topical nitrates (which act to relax the internal anal sphincter); however, at the moment only small studies have been performed, with promising results.

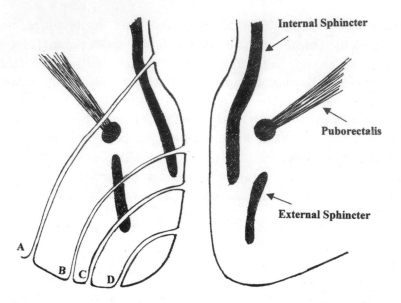

Figure 8.1. Perianal fistulae. Cross-section through the anal canal and lower rectum showing the normal anatomy on the right and the different types of fistulae on the left. (A) Pelvianal fistula; (B) high anal fistula; (C) low anal fistula; (D) subcutaneous anal fistula.

Fistula *in Ano*

A fistula is an abnormal connection between two epithelial surfaces [NB: A sinus is a blind-ending tract joing an epithelial surface to a cavity lined by granulation tissue (e.g. an abscess).]

A fistula *in ano* has an opening internally to the anal canal and another opening externally onto the skin. Most probably start as a perianal abscess, but occasionally they are due to Crohn's disease, carcinoma, radiotherapy or tuberculosis. They can be classified as "low" when they do not cross the sphincter muscles and "high" when they cross the sphincters. Low fistulae are usually treated by being laid open. This is achieved by inserting a metal probe into the fistula and incising through the tissue down onto the probe. The wound is allowed to heal from its depths upwards. This cannot be done with high fistulae, because the sphincters would be damaged, and so these fistulae may be treated with a seton. This is a wire or thread which is passed through the fistula track and is tied on the outside. It can then be gradually tightened so that over a period of weeks it cuts through to the surface, with the fistula healing by scar tissue behind it.

Goodsall's rule states that fistulae anterior to the anus usually open to the anus in a straight line whilst posterior ones usually have a curving track and open in the mid-line posteriorly.

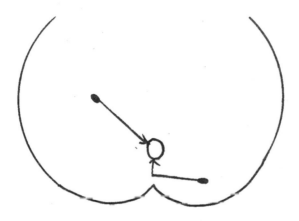

Figure 8.2. Goodsall's rule.

Rectal Prolapse

Rectal prolapse may be partial or complete. Partial prolapse is defined as involving the mucosa alone and obviously this rarely prolapses for more than a few centimetres. Complete prolapse involves prolapse of the full thickness of the rectum and can be much more sizable. It is most common in elderly females and presents with a mass that appears on or during defaecation. It may reduce spontaneously or require manual reduction and sometimes will present as a semiemergency as a prolapse which has become oedematous and ulcerated, producing pain and bleeding.

Rectal prolapse is usually associated with poor anal sphincter function. Initial treatment is to reduce the prolapse manually, but this will often be only a temporary solution. Because a prolapse may be treated by Phenol injection (to induce scarring) or by simple excision of the mucosa, but full thickness prolapse usually needs a full operation, such as an abdominal rectopexy (where the abdomen is entered and the rectum is stitched up, usually on to the sacrum, in order to prevent further prolapse) or a Delorme's procedure, in which the mucosa is excised and the rectal muscle plicated and then returned into the anal canal. A procedure known as a Thiersch tape or wire used to be employed. This consisted of passing a tape or wire around the anal canal subcutaneously in order to hold the prolapse inside. This operation has now been largely abandoned because of problems with recurrent prolapse or constipation.

Perianal Haematoma

A perianal haematoma is sometimes also called a thrombosed external haemorrhoid (which is a misnomer, as it is not actually a haemorrhoid). It is usually due to subcutaneous bleeding around the anal margin caused by the passage of constipated stool. It produces acute perianal pain which may be worsened by defaecation or movement. Examination will reveal a tense tender blue lump at the anal margin which can be simply treated by incision under local anaesthetic should the symptoms be too severe to be controlled by simple analgesia.

Anorectal Abscess

Anorectal or perianal abscesses are a common problem and are frequently seen as emergencies. They may either be perianal, ischiorectal or intermuscular (where they extend between the internal and external sphincters). Occasionally they represent spread from a pelvic abscess down to the perianal region. It is thought that there are two main reasons for the development of these abscesses. Firstly, they may develop from infection in an anal gland, which then turns into an abscess. These will usually have intestinal type organisms within them (e.g. *E. coli*). Others may develop from simple skin infections, such as an infected sebaceous gland or hair follicle, and are therefore more likely to contain staphylococci.

The patient will usually be complaining of a severe throbbing pain, worse on sitting, and may have signs of a fever, tachycardia, etc. The treatment is surgical drainage, packing and healing by secondary intention. The patient should be seen subsequently in the out-patient clinic to see if there is any evidence of an underlying fistula *in ano*, which occurs in up to 30% of patients.

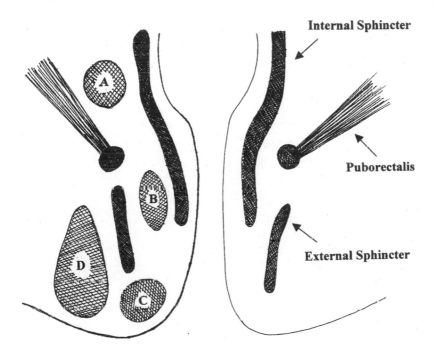

Figure 8.3. Perianal abscesses. (A) Pelvirectal abscess; (B) intersphinteric abscess; (C) perianal abscess; (D) ischiorectal abscess.

Pilonidal Abscess/Sinus

The word "pilonidal" comes from a Latin word meaning "nest of hair". A pilonidal abscess or sinus is usually found in the natal cleft. The exact aetiology is still not completely understood but they are thought to be an acquired rather than a congenital (as was once thought) condition. The hairs within the pilonidal cavity are thought to be hairs which have worked their way under the skin and not hairs growing within the sinus or abscess cavity. The condition is more common in people in their teenage and young adult years. It is more common in men than in women and, as one might expect, in those who are particularly hairy. It also seems to be more common in those whose occupation involves prolonged sitting, such as those who drive for a living.

The patient is usually unaware of the sinus until it becomes secondarily infected and presents as an abscess. Treatment of a pilonidal abscess is incision and drainage, followed by packing and healing by secondary intention. Later on a second procedure is needed to excise the sinus tract (which may extend for some distance away from the opening and which can be outlined by injection of methylene blue into the orifices of the sinuses at the time of surgery). If the excised area is small enough it may be possible to close the area primarily. Alternatively it may be necessary to leave the area open to heal by secondary intention.

Pilonidal disease has a significant tendency to recur even after apparently successful surgery. Patients should be encouraged to be scrupulous with their personal hygiene and to keep the area clean and dry and free from any loose hairs.

9

THE ACUTE ABDOMEN

It is unlikely that any cases of acute abdominal pain will be seen as clinical cases in the finals. This is simply because of the difficulty of arranging such cases in advance. However, cases who have had previous acute abdominal problems may be included as long cases and questions on acute abdominal conditions will be commonly found in written papers and vivas. Indeed, the examiners will often place great importance on candidates having a good knowledge of diagnosis and management in the acute abdomen, as they know that the subject will be of immediate relevance when the candidate takes up his general surgical house job.

The acute abdomen is usually defined as a case of abdominal pain with a short history (usually less than one week), presenting as an emergency with no history of trauma.

It is worth remembering, in answering questions, that such patients will usually be assessed in casualty departments and, as well as history and examination, simpler investigations such as blood tests and plain X-rays are likely to be all that is initially available. To a large extent the management of the acute abdomen is not, therefore, based on complex investigations but on clinical acumen.

Abdominal Pain

As with all pains, a certain number of features should be elicited, namely:

- Site (at onset and currently); see Figure 9.1.
- What is the nature of the pain (character, frequency, radiation)?
- How did the pain start and what has happened to it since?

- What relieves and what exacerbates the pain?
- Are there any associated symptoms?
- Have you ever had this before? / previous history.
- What do you think it is?

It is helpful to consider the underlying aetiology of the pain so as to try and classify types of acute abdominal pain further. In broad terms, pain in the acute abdomen is caused by one of the following:

(1) Pain due to inflammation (i.e. peritonitis).
(2) Pain due to obstruction of a hollow viscus (i.e. colic).
(3) Referred pain (e.g. pain referred from nerve root compression).
(4) Pain in a specific organ or mass (e.g. hepatitis).

Colic is defined as pain caused by obstruction of a hollow viscus and, in the context of the acute abdomen, may arise from obstruction of the small intestine, ureter, biliary system, colon, uterus or fallopian tubes and the appendix. When a hollow viscus with smooth muscle in its walls is obstructed, the smooth muscle contracts in peristaltic waves in an attempt to overcome the obstruction. These spasmodic contractions give rise to intermittent spasms of pain. The classical example is small bowel colic, where pain will come and grip the patient for a short period of time, be so severe as to double him up or make him cry out with pain, and will then wear off before another attack occurs, usually a few minutes later. Pain from viscera is usually not well localized and probably travels along the autonomic nerves which have no dermatomal distribution. The gut developed embryologiclly from midline structures and hence pain is generally referred to the midline. Fore-gut structures (oesophagus to second part duodenum) usually give rise to pain in the upper abdomen, mid-gut structures (second part duodenum to transverse colon) give rise to pain in the middle of the abdomen, and hind-gut structures give rise to pain in the lower abdomen. Thus small bowel colic is usually felt centrally, etc.

Peritonitis means inflammation of the peritoneum. In contrast to visceral pain, the parietal peritoneum is innervated by somatic nerves and hence pain is accurately localised to the site of inflammation. This type of pain is typically worse with movement, coughing or inspiration and therefore the patient lies still with shallow breaths (unlike colicky pain, where he moves about to try to get comfortable). Peritonitis is associated with guarding or rigidity of the abdominal muscles. There appear to be some differences in opinion as to the true definition of guarding and rigidity; however, most surgeons would agree that guarding is an involuntary (reflex) contraction of the abdominal muscles when the examining hand presses down over the inflamed area. It is sometimes difficult to differentiate true guarding from voluntary guarding, where the patient contracts his own abdominal muscles in anticipation of pain (especially seen in children). However, if you palpate the two sides of the abdomen at the same time while distracting the patient, you may find that the muscles appear tense on one side compared to the other. It is not really possible to do this voluntarily (where the two sides contract symmetrically) and hence this must be true guarding. If at rest the patient's abdominal musculature has an increased tone, then this is termed rigidity and is again due to underlying inflammation of the peritoneum. If peritonitis involves the whole abdomen, then the patient would typically present with a boardlike, rigid, tender abdomen with absent bowel sounds.

Examination of the Abdomen

Obviously it is always important to do a general examination of the patient. In particular, attention should be paid to signs of shock or dehydration as manifested by peripheral shut-down, clamminess, pallor, tachycardia and hypotension. One can often tell, just by looking at the patient, whether he is unwell. The typical patient with peritonitis looks pale and sweaty, with sunken eyes and a weak thready pulse, shallow breaths and little movement — as first described by Hippocrates thousands of years ago.

Introduce yourself to the patient, ask if he minds your examining him and if he has any pain. Lay him flat (one pillow) and adequately undress him (ideally from nipples to knees, but in the exam you should try to preserve the patient's dignity). On inspection of the abdomen (from the foot of the bed) observe for any obvious scars or masses, distension and the movement with respiration. You may find it easier in an exam situation to comment on your observations as you go along (unless you are confident you can present it all at the end). It is sometimes difficult to differentiate fat from distension (which can be due to flatus or fluid or foetus or faeces).

Next, hold the hand and look for any nail changes (e.g. clubbing), liver palms, etc., feel the pulse, look into the mouth for furring of the tongue and for dry mucous membranes, look into the eyes for jaundice or anaemia (pale conjunctiva), and swiftly feel the neck for any lymph nodes.

On palpation of the abdomen (make sure the hands are warm) kneel down to the patient's right, so that you are roughly level with him. The abdomen can be divided into theoretical regions as in Figure 9.1.

Starting at the furthest point from where he tells you the pain is, gently feel in each of these regions. This gives you a quick idea of any obvious masses or tender areas and whether the abdomen is soft. You should begin to think of what anatomical structures are under this area. Always look up at the patient's face (for grimacing). Next you can palpate a little deeper to build up on the findings of gentle palpation. Note if there is any guarding, rigidity or rebound. Rebound tenderness (most painful when the examining hand is removed) is not a good test, as it often causes the patient unnecessary pain and can give equivocal results. Tenderness on percussion is a more accurate and kinder way of assessing the same thing.

Examine the liver and spleen (starting in the right iliac fossa for both, with the patient inspiring each time you press in). In right upper quadrant abdominal pain, Murphy's test for cholecystitis is relevant, and if any masses or enlarged organs are palpated then the precise features need to be delineated. After palpation, percussion should be used before auscultation. Bowel sounds should be classified as being present (i.e. normal), absent (must listen for 3 min) or obstructive (high-pitched and tinkling).

Always finish your examination by palpating for an abdominal aortic aneurysm and check the hernial orifices and scrotum. A rectal examination

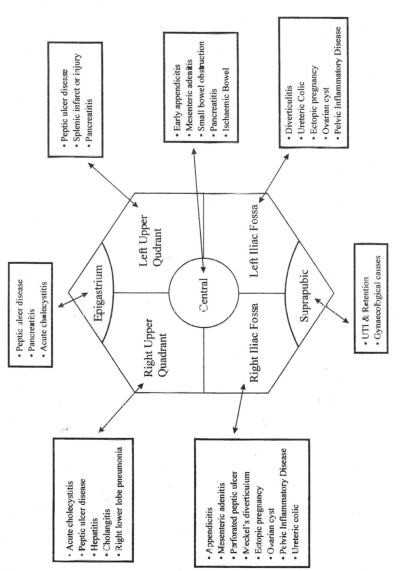

Figure 9.1. Areas of the abdomen. The boxes contain the possible diagnoses of pain in these regions.

is mandatory (although in an exam you usually just state that you would like to do it). The breast is really part of the abdominal examination, since if you were shown a case of ascites in the exam and you did not comment on the mastectomy scar, you would not receive any bonus points!

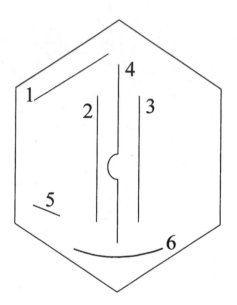

Figure 9.2. Abdominal incisions: (1) right subcostal or Kocher's incision; (2) right paramedian; (3) left paramedian; (4) mid-line; (5) gridiron (Lanz); (6) Pfannenstiel.

Acute Abdomen: Causes

(1) *Intestinal*

- Acute appendicitis
- Mesenteric adenitis
- Meckel's diverticulitis
- Perforated peptic ulcer
- Gastroenteritis

- Diverticulitis
  - perforated
  - nonperforated
- *Intestinal Obstruction*
  - strangulated hernia
  - adhesions

(2) *Hepatobiliary*

- Panreatitis
- Gallstones
  - biliary colic
  - cholecystitis
  - cholangitis
- Hepatitis

(3) *Vascular*

- Ruptured aortic aneurysm
- Mesenteric embolus/thrombosis
- Ischaemic colitis

(4) *Urological Causes*

- Renal colic
- Urinary infection
- Torsion of testicle
- Acute retention of urine

(5) *Gynaecological Causes*

- Ectopic pregnancy
- Ovarian cyst
  - torsion
  - ruptured
- Salpingitis
- Endometriosis
- Mittelschmerz

(6) *Medical Causes*

- Pneumonia/pleurisy
- Cardiac pain/pericarditis
- Herpes zoster
- Diabetes — ketoacidosis
- Neurological pain
- Hypercalcaemia
- Sickle cell crisis
- Syphilis/porphyria

Treatment of the Acute Abdomen

Most students learn each topic as it is laid out in the textbooks. However, in real life a patient does not present saying: "I have acute appendicitis," and neither does he always present with the classical textbook description. Instead most patients tend to present with a variety of vague symptoms and signs that do not point to any specific diagnosis. The acute abdomen is the best topic for highlighting this fact, because a patient who presents with epigastric pain and vomiting could be having pancreatitis, cholecystitis, a perforated peptic ulcer or just gastritis, and it may not be possible to differentiate on the history alone. The examination and simple investigations add further clues to help make a diagnosis, but still it may not be possible to make an absolute diagnosis initially and management may consist of simple treatment such as resuscitation, analgesia and a period of observation whilst further investigations are performed. In other cases, although a specific diagnosis is not made, exploratory laparotomy may be needed (i.e. in cases of generalised peritonitis).

As a student, making the wrong diagnosis is not that important, because there will always be a doctor available to correct you. As a doctor, however, you need to ask yourself "What if I am wrong?" with each decision made, since performing an appendicectomy on a patient with mesenteric adenitis is unlikely to be life-threatening; on the other hand, if you make a diagnosis of acute appendicitis in a female with right-sided pain without first performing a pregnancy test, then the surgeon may be left with an appendicectomy incision to deal with an ectopic pregnancy.

For example, let us say a 14-year-old girl presents with right iliac fossa pain and nausea. The possible causes of this are appendicitis, mesenteric adenitis, a UTI, an ectopic pregnancy or any other gynaecological problem, or even just wind. You should, therefore, ask not only the pertinent questions that point to a specific diagnosis but also the questions that will rule out the other diagnoses. Thus note the menstrual history and the history of the pain; for example, the pain of appendicitis usually starts centrally and moves to the right side after a few hours, whereas a torsion of an ovarian cyst gives a sudden onset of right iliac fossa pain. A UTI usually has associated urinary symptoms (frequency, dysuria and urgency).

Next, you derive further clues from the examination, looking for localised right iliac fossa tenderness or peritonism. Further clues are again derived from the simple investigations. A pregnancy test and urine dipstix and urgent microscopy must be performed to rule out an infection. A simple blood test such as a white cell count may help (although it is not that specific), and plain X-rays may give further clues (although not that helpful in this case, they would be if renal stones or bowel obstruction were on the differential).

At this point you may have narrowed the differential down to appendicitis, mesenteric adenitis or a gynaecological problem, but you still may not be exactly sure which it is. It is safe then to admit the patient, start IV fluids and carefully observe her with repeated examinations. If the pain and tenderness appear to settle, no further treatment may be necessary. However, if they persist, then it may be necessary to investigate the patient further. An ultrasound can be helpful, as it can visualise the ovaries and look for any free fluid. It may even show up an enlarged appendix. In this situation an ultrasound is very sensitive although not that specific, and even if it shows no abormality it does not rule out appendicitis. Another option is to perform a diagnostic laparoscopy where the organs are visualised directly via a laparascope. If the appendix is inflamed it could be removed laparascopically (if the surgeon has enough experience) or conversion to an open procedure can take place.

In a male with the same history, symptoms and signs there is not much else it can be apart from appendicitis and mesenteric adenitis, and if the pain did not settle after a period of observation many surgeons would agree that an appendicectomy was indicated without any further investigation.

If you are asked to write an essay on the acute abdomen, remember that whilst there are many causes of acute abdominal pain, most are relatively rare. Try to weight your answers to give the most prominence to the more common diagnoses. Obviously treatment depends on the specific diagnosis made, but it usually consists of resuscitation (oxygen, IV fluids, analgesia, etc.), admission for observation (nasogastric tubes, catheters, fluid balance, repeated examinations, etc.) or even an exploratory laparotomy.

10

BREAST SURGERY

EXAMINATION

Examination of the breast should be practised many times before finals. Breast cancer is very topical and frequently comes up in essays, vivas and long cases. Examination is difficult because it requires a lot of effort to make the patient, who undoubtedly will be anxious, feel at ease. You yourself may be even more nervous or embarrassed than the patient.

Inspection

Ask the patient to sit up either on the side of the bed or in a chair, exposing the upper half of her body. With her arms at her side observe for any obvious deformities (remember that the breasts are usually of slightly unequal size), skin dimpling, previous scars, inversion and/or eczema of the nipple. Then ask her to raise her arms above her head, helping to expose the lower parts of her breasts, which may make any deformities more obvious.

Then ask the patient to lie flat with arms by her side. Most surgeons have by this stage asked the patient to identify where she feels the lump is.

Always start with the normal breast first. Lift the arm, on the side you are about to examine, and place the hand above her head. This allows the breast tissue to spread out over the chest wall. Repeat the inspection as above.

Palpation

Divide the breast into five imaginary areas: the four quadrants and a central nipple area. Remember that the upper outer quadrant extends up into the axillary tail, and is the commonest site for malignancies. There is no correct place to start as long as you systematically examine all the areas.

Feel gently in each area by using the flat surface of the fingers of the hand. Feel for the consistency (i.e. nodularity), which may be the same throughout both breasts. Then, using the fingertips, you can examine a little more clearly any lumps you have identified. Examine the nipple and areola. If there is a history of discharge, by gently squeezing the ducts in this area you may be able to elicit a discharge from the nipple. Note its colour and whether it is from multiple ducts or, more worryingly, from a single duct.

Now repeat the examination of the opposite, affected breast. Remember that if you find a lump you should be thinking, as with any other lump, of its site, size, shape, colour, contour, consistency, temperature, tenderness, tethering, transilluminance, etc.

To assess if the lump is tethered more deeply, ask the patient to place her hands on her hips and push inwards. If there is deep fixity the deformity of the breast may be exaggerated.

Once you have examined the breast you must examine for lymphatic spread. Swiftly feel the neck and supraclavicular fossa, then move on to the axilla.

You must take the strain off pectoralis major and latissimus dorsi to allow proper examination of the axilla. Therefore, take the weight from her arm by holding it at the elbow, and asking her to relax and let the arm drop to the side. A hand poking about in the armpit is quite uncomfortable, so make sure you inform her of this before you start.

In the exam situation, before you finish the examination you should always say that you would also like to examine the chest, abdomen (feeling for the liver) and spinal column for evidence of metastatic spread, although in reality clinical examination does not usually pick up asymptomatic metastases.

BREAST CANCER

Breast cancer affects 1 in 12 women in the UK. It is quite likely that you will see a case in finals. Between the ages of 40 and 50 it is the main cause of death in women.

The incidence of breast cancer increases with increasing age, although the percentage of deaths due to breast cancer peaks around 40–50 and then falls off. This is probably due to the fact that older women die of other diseases before the breast cancer becomes significant. This can be shown diagrammatically:

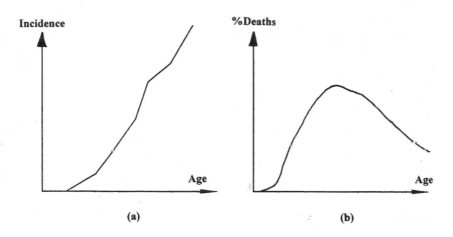

Figure 10.1. (a) incidence of breast cancer vs age; (b) per cent of deaths attributable to breast cancer vs age.

The risk factors for breast cancer are multiple, the most important being previous breast cancer or a family history.

Family History

There is certainly a significant genetic contribution predisposing women to breast cancer, probably inherited as an autosomal dominant trait with limited penetrance. In other words, you may inherit the gene from your father or mother, yet you or your mother may never get breast cancer. Up to 10% of breast cancers are due to a genetic predisposition. So far several breast cancer genes have been identified, such as the BRCA1 and BRCA2 genes (on the long arms of chromosome 17 and 13 respectively).

In many families affected by breast cancer, an increased prevalence of ovarian, colon and other cancers has also been noticed. These are thought to be related to the same inherited mutation. Breast cancers that are due to a genetic mutation tend to strike women at a young age.

If a young women has a first degree relative who was affected by breast cancer before the age of 50, then her risk of developing breast cancer at a young age is doubled. If, however, this first degree relative developed breast cancer after the age of 50, then her risk is increased only slightly.

Exposure to Oestrogens

Early menarche, late menopause, nulliparity and late age of first conception, all increase the risk for breast cancer.

The Oral Contraceptive Pill

Use of the oral contraceptive pill (OCP) for greater than four years in younger women before their first pregnancy has been shown in some studies to increase the risk of premenopausal breast cancer. Women who use the OCP for short periods to space pregnancies are at no increased risk.

Hormone Replacement Therapy

The majority of studies show that the use of hormone replacement therapy (HRT) for menopausal symptoms is associated with an increased risk of breast cancer, and use for greater than ten years significantly increases the risk. Recently published studies show that the addition of progestins to the oestrogen preparations in order to protect against endometrial cancer in fact compounds the risk of breast cancer.

The increased risk of breast cancer must be balanced against the benefits in terms of reduction of morbidity from ischaemic heart disease and osteoporosis, and most nowadays would advocate the use of HRT for somewhere between five and ten years.

Previous benign breast disease. Severe atypical epithelial hyperplasia significantly increases the risk for breast cancer. Most other forms of benign breast disease have no role in causation of breast cancer.

Radiation, geography and lifestyle are other risk factors. Obesity in premenopausal women is associated with a decreased incidence of breast cancer, whereas in postmenopausal women, obesity doubles their risk. This may have something to do with peripheral conversion of oestrogens.

A low socioeconomic group, a diet high in saturated fats and high alcohol intake have all been linked with an increased risk of breast cancer. The associations are likely to be compounded and the true relationship is unclear. Smoking has been advocated as a risk factor; however, the largest studies performed have shown that smoking does *not* increase the risk of breast cancer.

Management and the Clinic

The ideal breast clinic has a multidisciplinary team which includes a consultant breast surgeon, a specialist breast care nurse, a coordinator (usually a secretary) who brings all the results together, together with an experienced radiologist, a histopathologist and a cytologist.

In some centres these clinics run very efficiently, with the time taken from presentation to diagnosis amounting to only a few days, and occasionally hours.

Patients arrive at the clinic via two routes. Either the lady has an incidental finding on screening mammography in an otherwise asymptomatic lump, or she notices a breast lump and is referred to the clinic via her GP. If the GP is concerned, the lady is usually seen very quickly by the clinic.

Any woman presenting with a breast lump undergoes three things, sometimes called *triple assessment.*

Triple Assessment

(1) A careful history and examination.
(2) An imaging technique.
(3) Fine needle aspiration.

When the patient arrives at the clinic she undergoes triple assessment. In most of the good clinics she can return that evening to the clinic to get the results of her tests.

(1) In your *history* you must ask about all of the above risk factors for breast cancer and then obtain a history of the lump (see page 8).

Do not forget to ask about menarche, parity and age at birth of children, menstrual cycle and regularity, age of menopause, use of medication including OCP and HRT, family history, etc.

The history will give you many hints as to the likely diagnosis; remember that cysts can appear overnight, and they together with other forms of benign breast disease tend to be related to the menstrual cycle. The woman may have had previous cysts drained by a surgeon.

Pain is not a typical symptom of breast cancer. If the patient complains of a nipple discharge, you must ask for the colour, as blood-stained discharges are more worrying than a clear or milky one. When examining you must attempt to elicit whether this is from a single duct or many ducts.

With regard to breast cancer, the patient that is worrying is the one presenting classically with many risk factors for breast cancer and a single lump, in a single area of a single breast.

(2) *What techniques are there for imaging?*

Mammography

This is performed in the radiology department and may be quite uncomfortable for the patient. The breast is compressed between two plates. The one above the breast is made of clear perspex and the one below contains the X-ray plate. The X-rays are directed through the compressed breast onto the X-ray plate.

Craniocaudal and oblique views can be obtained, looking for obvious dense masses or just spicules of microcalcification.

The breast is relatively radiodense below the age of 35, and so higher doses of radiation need to be used in order to get a suitable image. Ultrasound is therefore the investigation of choice for women below the age of 35. Some women may have both investigations performed.

Ultrasound

This is painless (unless the area is very tender) and cheap to perform; however, it needs experienced operators and analysis is subjective.

Ultrasound is excellent for showing up cysts which are transparent and rounded; solid lesions also show up and are especially suspicious if the edge is irregular or distorted.

(3) *Fine needle aspiration*

Often called fine needle aspiration cytology (FNAC), this is a simple procedure that can be performed in the breast clinic; however, at some centers it is performed in the cytology or radiology department.

A needle is placed into the breast lump, and a solid or liquid material is aspirated using a syringe. If the lump is impalpable it may need to be attempted under ultrasound or mammographic guidance.

The sample is smeared onto a microscope slide. It is then fixed (usually in air) and stained as appropriate.

The results of this test are placed in five categories, scored from 1 to 5. A score of 1 means an inadequate sample (for example, mostly fat cells were obtained), a score of 2 is normal, and a score of 5 is diagnostic of malignancy. It therefore follows that a score of 3 or 4 is somewhere between these extremes, with atypical features, but that still may be normal.

This procedure may also be the treatment for benign breast cysts. If you can fully aspirate the cyst until the lump disappears and there is no blood staining the aspirate, no further treatment may be needed for the lady (providing triple assessment has been performed). If, however, the lump persists or if the fluid is blood-stained (which could indicate a papillary tumour), then the lady should undergo further assessment.

Remember that a cytological diagnosis only tells you if it is benign or malignant (based on the presence of features such as abnormal mitoses, increased nuclear-to-cytoplasmic ratio, etc.); it cannot differentiate between an *in situ* and an invasive cancer.

TRUCUT BIOPSY

If the FNA is unhelpful or a definitive tissue diagnosis is required, then one can opt for one of two choices in the next stage of diagnosis: either the lump is excised or a trucut biopsy is performed. This allows a histological diagnosis to be made on the lump. In contrast to cytology, this can tell you if the cancer is invasive or not. The sample then gets sent to histology and allows a diagnosis to be made and treatment options to be decided. The patient returns to the clinic after a few days for the result.

A trucut biopsy can be done either at the clinic or on the ward. An aseptic technique is used under local anaesthetic. The needle is essentially large, with a sheath that slides over it, to allow a core of tissue to be sampled from the breast lump.

Both FNA's and trucuts may need to be performed under ultrasound or mammographic guidance if the lump is very small or impalpable.

TYPES OF BREAST CANCER

All breast cancers arise from the terminal duct lobular unit. They can be divided into invasive or noninvasive (*in situ*) cancers. If the cancer is confined within the basement membrane of the ducts and lobules, then it is by definition an *in situ* or noninvasive cancer.

Carcinomas *in Situ*

These are categorized by the histological pattern and the cell type. The pathologist classifies them as either high or low grade. The high grade ductal carcinoma *in situ* (DCIS) tumours have a much worse prognosis and are much more likely to go on to become invasive. One characteristic of DCIS is that there is calcification within the tumour allowing it to be picked up on screening mammograms.

The commonest form of noninvasive cancer is DCIS, accounting for about 20% of screen-detected and 3% of symptomatic cancers.

Before screening came about this condition was not really clinically relevant, and the truth is we do not really now what percentage of women with this condition will go on to develop invasive breast cancer. The natural course of these cancers has been described either in women who declined treatment or in those where disease was missed. Somewhere between 20 and 30% of these patients developed invasive breast cancer in the same breast over the subsequent 10–18 years. This means that we are treating four out of five women for a process that would never develop into invasive cancer.

Lobular carcinoma *in situ* is the other type of noninvasive cancer. It is much rarer and tends to be multifocal. It is therefore usually managed by close observation.

Invasive Cancer

Histological classification of invasive breast cancer is usually into those of the *special type* and those of *no special type*. "Special type" means that the tumour displays recognizable patterns of growth and cellular morphology.

For example, if the tumour's appearance is papillary or tubular, then since we can recognize this, we classify it as a special type. If, on the other hand, we cannot demonstrate distinct appearances, then the tumour is classified as being of the *nonspecial type*. The relevance of this is that tumours of the special type usually have a much better prognosis than those of no special type.

There is a condition called Paget's disease of the nipple, which presents as a unilateral red, eczematous lesion of the nipple that may ulcerate and bleed. This represents invasion of the nipple by malignant cells which reach the surface via spread along the breast ducts. The malignant cells come from an area of underlying DCIS. By the time of presentation there may also be an invasive cancer in the breast. Treatment is usually mastectomy.

STAGING

There are several systems used to stage breast cancer; unfortunately, none is particularly well suited to this disease, and they are therefore a crude way of categorizing patients.

If there is no evidence of distal metastases, then the presence or absence of axillary metastases (lymph nodes) is the best prognostic indicator of survival.

The tumour, node, metastases (TNM) staging system is now used for most cancers. It is based on the tumour size (T), the presence of metastases in lymph nodes (N) and the existence of distant metastases (M). The clinically assessed TNM stage can be adjusted once the pathologist has analysed the specimen (TNM_p).

TNM Staging System:

T_1 — tumour < 2 cm
T_2 — tumour 2–5 cm
T_3 — tumour > 5 cm
T_4 — direct extension to skin or chest wall

N_0 — no palpable lymph nodes (LN's)

N_1 — Mobile LN's on same side
N_2 — Fixed LN's on same side
N_3 — supraclavicular or infraclavicular LN's or arm lymphoedema

M_0 — no evidence of distant metastases
M_1 — distant metastases present

The International Union Against Cancer (UICC) system incorporates the TNM system (e.g. Stage I = $T_1N_0M_0$ and Stage IV = $T_{1-4}N_{0-3}M_1$) and divides the cancers into early (Stages I & II) and advanced (Stages III & IV) breast cancers. This staging system is used in most of the breast cancer treatment trials together with the histological grading and pathological node status.

You do not need to learn these staging systems but should have an understanding of how they work and their role.

Remember that *staging* is a clinical entity, whereas *grading* is what the histopathologist classifies according to the cell type and morphology. High grade or poorly differentiated tumours carry the worst prognosis.

When a patient is on the ward and you as the houseman are clerking her in, it is your duty to help complete the staging process. You should perform a full blood count, liver function tests and a chest X-ray on every patient with breast cancer. In those with advanced (Stages III & IV) cancer you should organize an ultrasound of the liver and a bone scan. Some departments insist on performing the latter tests at any stage of breast cancer; however, in those with early breast cancer, with normal blood and normal CXR, the ultrasound and bone scan have a low pick-up of metastases.

SPREAD

Like any other cancer, spread is by:

(1) *Direct extension* — to adjacent structures.
(2) *Lymphatics* — of the breast are essentially along its blood supply. The majority travel along the tributaries of the axillary vessels to the axilla, although a small proportion go medially and deeply to

the internal mammary nodes. Blockage of the lymphatics by an infiltrating cancer leads to oedema of the overlying skin, which becomes pitted by the adherence of the sweat ducts and hair follicles, leading to the appearance of an orange peel, and is hence called peau d'orange).

(3) *Blood spread* — especially to the liver, lungs and bones (axial skeleton, which has red bone marrow, such as the skull, spine, ribs and pelvis). Lobular carcinomas also tend to spread to the gastrointestinal tract. Initially micrometastases travel in the blood and seed at various sites in the body; whether they grow there depends on many other tumour and host factors.

(4) *Transcoelomic spread* — for example pleural seedings leading to a malignant pleural effusion.

TREATMENT OF BREAST CANCER

All you need to have for finals is a broad understanding of the principles behind the treatment of breast cancer. There are many varying opinions as to the correct treatment for a particular lesion. The examiner may not agree with your treatment but cannot fail you if you offer a sensible and acceptable option. Remember to stress the importance of involving the patient in the decision making process.

The information upon which we now base our treatments has come from clinical trials. Two of the most substantial facts about breast cancer have come from clinical trials, namely we know that breast conservation surgery with radiotherapy is as good as mastectomy and that adjuvant chemotherapy prolongs survival.

The main aim in the surgical treatment of breast cancer is the control of local disease. Surgery has no major role in improving survival. If microscopic metastases have occurred by the time of presentation, then no matter what operation you do you cannot alter survival. You can, however, stop the local spread, which is what causes the major morbidity (such as a fungating tumour within the breast or axilla). On the other hand, you can alter survival (*mortality*) by adjuvant systemic treatment, and we will cover this later.

To help order your thought process, try dividing your answer into the treatment of the breast, the treatment of the axilla and the treatment of micrometastases.

Treatment of the Breast

This can range from a lumpectomy, wide local excision (a lumpectomy with wider margins), to mastectomy. Nowadays we try to perform conservative surgery, which for malignant tumours usually means wide local excision (WLE). The indications for a simple mastectomy are if the lump is too large to remove without good cosmetic result, if the nipple is involved or if the disease is multifocal. Obviously you should use your common sense here, since a 2 cm lump in a small breast will be too big to do a WLE, but if a woman has very large breasts and the lump is peripheral then you may be able to get away with doing a WLE. At the operation a drain is usually placed into the wound to prevent a collection, and it is removed when the amount of draining begins to tail off, usually after a day or two.

In the past some patients had a radical mastectomy, but no one performs it these days as it is of no increased benefit. You may, however, see a case in finals of a lady 15 years after radical mastectomy. If the examiner takes you to see an elderly patient with a mastectomy scar and asks you to tell if this was a simple or a radical mastectomy, he expects you to test for the presence of the pec major muscle, finding it absent with weakness on the affected side, as this would have been removed in a radical procedure.

Malignant tumours that undergo WLE should be followed by radiotherapy to the breast and chest wall, as this improves local control. A study is currently underway looking at the need for radiotherapy in small, well-differentiated tumours, which may show that women with these tumours do not need radiotherapy.

If the lump is impalpable (usually picked up by screening mammography), then stereotactic localization is usually performed under mammographic control. A needle is placed into the area of microcalcification. The patient goes to theatre and has the area containing the needle and a surrounding margin excised. While the patient is still on the operating table the sample goes back (with the needle in it) to mammography, and it is re-X-rayed to ensure that the entire area of calcification has been excised.

In some circumstances a *frozen section* is needed. This is where the lump is removed and taken to the lab while the patient is still on the operating table, and the lump is frozen and sliced, and looked at under the microscope. The pathologist then rings the surgeon in theatre to report the result. If it is invasive then the surgeon goes on to treat the axilla in the same operation. This would be used, for example, if no definitive diagnosis had been reached with the triple assessment. To give an example, let us say the patient has a suspicious lump on mammography, the FNAC was C5, implying malignancy, but the trucut was unhelpful (just fat was picked up); then we know that this is a malignant lesion, but we do not know if it is an *in situ* or an invasive cancer. There are, therefore, several options for the surgeon: either the lump can be excised, and if the histology is invasive then a second operation on the axilla will be needed; or a frozen section will allow the surgeon to decide whether to go on and operate on the axilla in the same operation. This delays the procedure by about 20 min, but saves the need for a second operation. On the other hand many surgeons would perform axillary surgery without prior knowledge of any histology and without a frozen section either, basing this decision on the cytology result alone.

Treatment of the Axilla

There are about 28 lymph nodes in the axilla, but there are sometimes more. The presence of involved axillary lymph nodes is the single best predictor of survival from breast cancer. Treating the axilla does not affect survival. The theory is that distant micrometastases could have occurred by the time of presentation and it is these that will eventually kill the patient; hence, removing the axillary nodes will do nothing to prevent this.

The aim of treating the axilla is twofold: in order to stage the patient, allowing decisions to be made about further treatment such as chemotherapy (which may alter survival); and to prevent axillary recurrence.

The choices for treating a lady with breast cancer are to leave the axilla alone, to take a sample of lymph nodes or to clear the axilla.

Axillary sampling involves taking four separate lymph nodes from the axilla (the surgeon decides which nodes look like they may be affected). Studies have shown that these four nodes have good predictive value as to whether the other nodes in the axilla are affected.

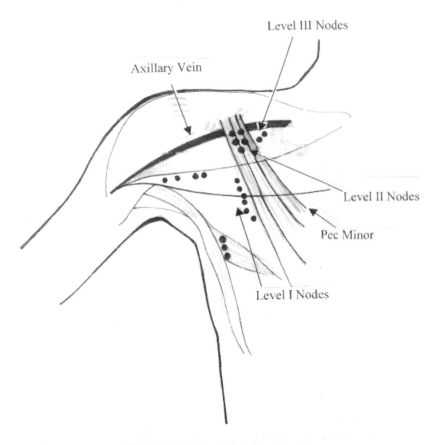

Figure 10.2. The axillary lymph nodes.

The alternative is to remove as many nodes as possible, causing as little damage to structures within the axilla as possible. Attempting to remove all the axillary lymph nodes is called axillary clearance; this is, however, technically more difficult and has a higher rate of complications such as nerve damage and lymphoedema. The lymph nodes are situated at different levels in the axilla. They are below the axillary vein and are described in relation to the pectoralis minor muscle. Those lateral to pec minor are at level I. Level II nodes sit behind pec minor. Level III nodes are medial to pec minor. Ideally, to clear the axilla one would have to remove nodes up to level III, and some surgeons always try to do this if a diagnosis of invasive cancer has been made.

However, if the surgeon opts to sample nodes from the axilla and finds that the histology confirms that they are affected, then he is left with a tough clinical decision. This is because there may be other affected nodes in the axilla which could develop into a compressive or fungating lesion at a later date, which can be devastating to the patient and very difficult to treat. Some surgeons would perform a second operation to clear the axilla. Others would advocate radiotherapy to the axilla. It is inadvisable to do both to the same axilla, due to the high rates of complications. A third option is to adopt a wait-and-see policy, following the patient up closely in the clinic, checking for evidence of recurrence and dealing with it only if it occurs.

The treatment of the axilla stirs up much debate, and really more clinical trials are needed to define the optimal treatment for the axilla.

Treatment of Micrometastases

By the time of presentation, micrometastases may have occurred, which are not usually picked up by our normal diagnostic techniques. We thus treat anyone likely to have metastases by adjuvant systemic treatment.

The difficulty is deciding which patients will benefit, taking into account the side effects they have to go through in the process.

Let us come off this subject for a moment to talk about hormone receptors. When the histopathologist analyses the breast lump, he can test for oestrogen and progesterone receptors. Hormone-receptor-positive patients tend to have a better prognosis and are more likely to respond to adjuvant treatment.

Adjuvant treatment is either chemotherapy or hormonal manipulation.

Adjuvant chemotherapy is used for young women (premenopausal) with positive lymph nodes or those with large primary tumours or those of an aggressive grade even if the lymph nodes are negative (as these patients have a worse prognosis). The drugs used are usually a combination of cyclophosphamide and fluorouracil, together with methotrexate or doxyrubicin (adriamycin), and are given as a course of treatments over a period of months. A large meta-analysis in 1992 showed that these regimens produce a 20% increase in survival in premenopausal women with axillary lymph node involvement (but without overt metastatic disease). A postmenopausal woman with an aggressive cancer may also require chemotherapy. The mechanism of action of these agents is thought to be a combination of ovarian ablation (hence reducing oestrogen levels) and direct attack of the tumour cells.

Hormonal treatment such as the tablet tamoxifen has been shown to increase the disease-free survival in postmenopausal women. Tamoxifen is both weakly oestrogenic and an oestrogen receptor (ER) antagonist. It is thought to act by disrupting the message generated when oestrogen binds to its receptor.

About 60% of ER-positive patients respond to hormonal manipulation, whereas only about 10% of ER-negative patients respond. Therefore, all postmenopausal women with ER-positive breast cancer are started on tamoxifen. Some would advocate that it should be given to all postmenopausal women. However, it does have side effects (menopausal symptoms and increased risk of endometrial cancer) and others may argue that with only a 10% chance of response in ER-negative women, these side effects might outweigh the benefits.

If a young women has a small tumour which is ER-positive, then one can offer tamoxifen. This has been shown also to reduce the incidence of tumours of the opposite breast by about 15%, but one must always bear in mind the pros and cons when considering its use. It is therefore not indicated in ER-negative young patients or those who go on to have chemotherapy.

Sometimes chemotherapy is given preoperatively if the lady has a large tumour, in the hope that it will shrink before excision. This is called neo-adjuvant chemotherapy.

Treatment of Advanced Breast Cancer

It is important that you understand the difference between advanced (Stages II & III) breast cancer and widespread metastatic disease. In advanced breast cancer the disease has spread locally but there is no evidence of any overt metastases. Patients often undergo surgery, which is usually a mastectomy, and they may be given radiotherapy as well and also chemotherapy. A surgical or chemical (e.g. Zoladex) oophorectomy can also be performed, to reduce the circulating oestrogens. Unfortunately, we do not know at present what the best treatment strategy is for advanced disease, since trials so far have shown that treatment with all of these modalities up front does not appear to decrease mortality any more than in patients who are treated sequentially with, say, surgery and radiotherapy initially, chemotherapy and/or oophorectomy then being administered if they appear to get a recurrence at follow-up.

Treatment of Widespread Metastatic Disease

If at the time of presentation a woman has distant metastases, then treatment goals are entirely different. The main aim here is to produce effective control of symptoms with minimal side effects. After all, the average period of survival after diagnosis of metastatic disease is only 18–24 months. In such people chemotherapy is usually not indicated unless the patient is symptomatic from the metastases (such as a pleural effusion). This is mainly because of the side effects that you will put the patient through in order to achieve only a small period of remission. In symptomatic patients, the overall response to chemotherapy is about 50%, with a median time to relapse of about 6–10 months.

Symptomatic treatment is important for these patients. Bony metastases can be treated with analgesia and radiotherapy. Malignant pleural effusions (diagnosed by cytology of the aspirate) can be treated by aspiration or drainage and often installation of bleomycin or tetracyclines into the pleural space (pleurodesis).

Surgical treatment for a cancer in these patients is advisable only if the lesion is ulcerating, fungating or very unsightly, and in this case it is called a toilet operation. There is no point operating on a breast lump if the patient is going to die from the metastases before the lump becomes symptomatic.

Radiotherapy

In the past mastectomy was a common operation for breast cancer. However, clinical trials that compared WLE and radiotherapy to mastectomy found that the results were almost equal after long term follow-up.

All women who have a WLE which is shown to be an invasive cancer receive irradiation to the affected breast and chest wall as an out-patient (usually given as a course over several weeks). Radiotherapy to the axilla is instituted less commonly these days, due to the complications.

Radiotherapy is sometimes used on a breast affected by DCIS, and studies looking at the role of radiotherapy in DCIS are underway.

The other use of radiotherapy is the treatment of localised bone pain that is due to metastases.

We realize that the above sounds very complex and so we have tried to summarize the treatment options in a simple way, by highlighting three broad patient groups (note that we have divided each section into treatment of the breast, treatment of the axilla, etc.):

(1) ***Treatment of DCIS*** (usually asymptomatic and picked up by screening mammography)

Breast — WLE, maybe under stereotactic guidance, and if the margins are clear and the tumour is small and not of an aggressive grade, then no further treatment is necessary.

If the margins are not clear, re-excise and treat as above.

If the DCIS is extensive, involving large areas of the breast or is multifocal, then the usual treatment is mastectomy. Some experienced surgeons perform bilateral subcutaneous mastectomies with immediate breast reconstruction. It is ironic that most invasive cancers are treated with a breast conservation, whereas a woman with widespread *in situ* carcinoma who may or may not go on to become invasive, is treated with a mastectomy.

If the lesions are extensive or the tumour is of an aggressive grade, then radiotherapy to the affected breast may improve the outcome.

Axilla — If the lesion is DCIS, which by definition has not invaded the basement membrane, then *no* axillary treatment is necessary.

(2) *A young (premenopausal) woman with invasive breast cancer*

Breast — WLE if possible; radiotherapy is then given to the remaining breast and chest wall. If the lesion is central, or very large in a small breast, then simple mastectomy is performed.

If the lesion is large (> 4 cm) and we know that it is ER-positive (from the FNA or trucut), a course of chemotherapy or tamoxifen may be used preoperatively, which may cause regression and shrinkage of the tumour, allowing breast-conserving treatment.

Axilla — Sampling or clearance (to help stage and prevent axillary recurrence; no effect on survival).

Micrometastatic spread — If axillary lymph nodes are positive or the tumour is large or of an aggressive histological grade, adjuvant chemotherapy is given.

If the patient has a small tumour that is ER-positive with negative lymph nodes, then tamoxifen could be considered.

(3) *An older (postmenopausal) woman with invasive breast cancer*

Breast and axilla — As for the younger woman.

Micrometastatic spread — If ER-positive, the patient should be on tamoxifen. If ER-negative, discuss with the patient the pros and cons of using tamoxifen.

If the tumour is very aggressive or there is extensive lymph node involvement, the patient may be offered chemotherapy.

Remember that if a lady in her nineties presents with a breast cancer, one option would be to offer just tamoxifen or radiotherapy and hence avoid surgery altogether. It is always advisable in the management of breast cancer to be honest and open when discussing a patient's treatment, involving her in the decision. After all the patient may wish for you to do absolutely nothing.

PROGNOSIS

The prognosis of a breast cancer patient depends on many factors, including stage, histological type and grade (especially presence of vascular invasion). The single best indicator is, however, the presence of axillary metastases. The number of involved nodes is directly correlated with survival.

As we have also mentioned, the absence of hormone receptors implies a poorer prognosis.

Some centres can analyse the tumour for the expression of the proto-oncogene erb B2 (which produces epidermal growth factor receptors). Patients with lymph node positive tumours that express erbB2 have a particularly poor prognosis and respond poorly to systemic treatment.

Some centres have developed their own formula, combining multiple independent variables to predict the prognosis. The Nottingham Prognostic Index (NPI), for example, incorporates tumour size, node status and histological grade. The NPI divides patients into good, intermediate and poor prognostic groups. The good prognostic group has a survival rate of approximately 90% at 5 years, whereas the poor prognistic group has about 25% survival at 5 years.

SCREENING

Mortality can be reduced by up to 30% in women who attend screening. In 1986 the Forest Report was published, which looked at the New York and Swedish screening programmes and made recommendations for the use of screening in the UK. The recommendations were that women between 50 and 65 should be invited every three years for a single oblique mammogram. The programme was implemented; however, most units now perform two views on the first screen to reduce the number of recalls. Each subsequent screen is just one oblique view.

If any abnormality is picked up in the screening mammogram, then the patient is recalled for subsequent views.

About 60 cancers per 10 000 attendees are picked up in the British screening programme.

For finals you need to be able to talk about any screening programme (generalized topic), namely that the disease is significant, that treatment is available and effective and the outcome can be affected, and that the test is simple, cheap, acceptable, unambiguous, with high specificity and sensitivity, etc.

Breast self-examination has been shown to have no effect on reducing mortality.

Regarding breast cancer you should think about the following points:

• The test (mammography) is expensive, requiring highly trained radiologists, and at best detects only 95% of breast cancers.
• Many women who are recalled are put through unnecessary investigations and worries (about two-thirds of women recalled are subsequently shown to have no cancer).
• Screen-detected cancers are more likely to be *in situ* than symptomatic cancers — are we, therefore, treating women who would never go on to develop invasive cancer? The fact that screening has reduced mortality from breast cancer suggests not.
• How frequently should women have a screening mammogram? In the UK we invite women every three years, because this is cost-effective. However, studies from other countries suggest that two

years or less is more appropriate for picking up interval cancers (cancers presenting between screenings).

- How many views — one or two? Will two views detect more cancers? There are no convincing data to confirm this. Remember, women would receive double the radiation exposure.
- Should we stop screening at age 65? After all, the incidence of breast cancer continues to rise with increasing age.

RECONSTRUCTIVE SURGERY

After having a mastectomy the woman may feel mutilated and suffer devastating emotional turmoil; for this reason she should be counselled preoperatively. The specialist breast care nurse plays a large part in this. Reconstructive surgery should therefore be available to any woman who requests it.

In the past, before the advent of screening, many women underwent radical mastectomies requiring quite extensive reconstructive techniques. Nowadays, with the emphasis being on breast-conserving surgery, reconstruction has been made easier.

Reconstruction can be carried out either by immediate placement of a prosthesis, or by using a tissue expander or a musculocutaneous flap.

The advent of the silastic (silicone) prosthesis has allowed good cosmetic results. It is usually placed below the pectoralis major muscle (as opposed to cosmetic breast augmentation, where the prosthesis is usually placed above the muscle — as there is still breast tissue), either directly or after a period of tissue expansion. This involves placing a plastic or silicone bag into the region and filling it up with saline periodically over a period of weeks, until the ideal size is achieved; this allows stretching of the skin and muscle. It can later be replaced with a silicone implant, or in some types just the valve mechanism can be removed, leaving the prosthesis *in situ*.

The musculocutaneous flaps are segments of muscle with their overlying skin that are transferred from one region to cover a defect in another. The blood supply to the skin usually comes from arteries that supply the muscle beneath, and hence moving the entire segment from one region to another often leads to avascular necrosis. Therefore, the segment is either rotated or tunnelled from one region to another, allowing the vascular pedicle supplying the segment to remain intact. The defect created by this flap can then be closed primarily or by using a skin graft. The commonest flaps include the latissimus dorsi musculocutaneous flap, which is tunnelled across to the front. Another example takes skin and muscle from just below the breast (i.e. the rectus abdominis muscle), called the transverse rectus abdominis myocutaneous (TRAM) flap. These techniques tend to be performed by those with expertise in the field of plastic surgery. Free flaps are a more advanced plastics technique where the entire musculocutaneous flap is removed together with its feeding blood supply and resited on to the breast. The blood supply is then reanastomosed to vessels in this region by microsurgical anastomotic techniques.

Delayed reconstruction has the advantage of letting the patient live with the scar of a mastectomy for a short while, so that once reconstruction is finished the end result, which will not be perfect, will be more acceptable. The nipple is quite a problem in reconstruction, and often requires transplanting skin from other darker regions such as the labia, or having the colour tattooed on later, or even the need for a false nipple.

A bilateral subcutaneous mastectomy with immediate insertion of a prosthesis is sometimes performed for extensive DCIS.

BENIGN BREAST DISEASE

The anatomy of the normal breast consists mainly of fibrous and fatty tissue. The areolar glands are typical sebaceous glands, separated by fibrous septa into lobules. Arising from the glands are between 15 and 20 lactiferous ducts that converge on the nipple.

All of the above tissues undergo cyclical proliferation and regression under the influence of hormones between puberty and menopause. It is normal, therefore, for the breasts to change in size, glandularity or nodularity with one's menstrual period.

One can look at benign breast disease as a spectrum of conditions ranging from the above normal changes to, say, the formation of huge cysts in the breast. If the whole lobule hypertrophies with a predominance of fibrous tissue, then a fibroadenoma (breast mouse) develops. This commonly presents as a solitary mobile lump in a younger woman. Fibroadenosis (also known as fibrocystic disease), on the other hand, is similar but affects all of the components of the breast rather than just the fibrous tissue and leads to diffuse lumpiness without one discreet lump, and tends to present in slightly older women (aged 35–45) with cyclical pain. Breast cysts are another form of fibroadenosis, where fluid-filled spaces predominate, and are common in premenopausal women.

Benign breast disease is not a predisposing cause of cancer [except for severe epithelial hyperplasia (epitheliosis)].

All patients who present to the clinic with a lump undergo triple assessment to rule out malignancy. If all of the tests on a lump suggest the diagnosis to be a fibroadenoma, then the patient and the surgeon are left with two options: either to leave the lump alone and simply follow the patient in the clinic or to excise it as a lumpectomy (this can be performed as a day case). The lump can, however, recur.

Traumatic fat necrosis is a condition where fat cells burst after trauma and cause an inflammatory reaction with giant cells and fibrosis. This presents with a hard lump that mimics breast cancer. It is a harmless condition but needs to be investigated to rule out cancer.

MASTALGIA

Breast pain (mastalgia) can be divided into two main subtypes: cyclical (related to the menstrual cycle and accounting for two-thirds of patients) and noncyclical (one-third). It is normal for a woman to feel some pain and fullness of the breasts a few days before her period.

Women with *cyclical mastalgia* suffer severe painful breasts from mid-cycle onwards. The pains often resolve on menstruation. *Noncyclical mastalgia* affects slighltly older women and has no relationship to the menstrual cycle. The aetiology of mastalgia is uncertain.

The type and severity of mastalgia can be assessed by the use of a breast pain record chart, which is a form of diary where pain is logged daily as severe, mild or absent over a period of a few months.

A careful history must be taken and a clinical examination performed to exclude any lumps (which should be investigated if present).

Treatment is essentially an explanation (that the cause is probably hormonal) and reassurance that there is no evidence of any malignancy. In most cases this is all that is needed; however, in the remaining cases, where the pain continues to interfere with the patient's lifestyle and sexual relationships, other treatments may be necessary.

Evening primrose oil (high dose gamolenic acid) helps in some cases (and may work by replacing certain essential fatty acids missing in these patients) but needs to be tried for at least four months. If it fails, danazol or bromocriptine can be tried, but these have other side effects. Recent reports suggest that tamoxifen can help in some cases but is not yet licensed for this in the UK. The oral contraceptive pill does not alleviate the pain of cyclical mastalgia.

In the case of noncyclical mastalgia (NCM), it is important first to rule out any causes of referred pain such as cardiac, chest or cervical spine pathology. A firm supportive bra worn all day and night and a course of nonsteroidal anti-inflammatories may improve symptoms. If these fail then the above treatments for cyclical mastalgia may be tried. In some patients with NCM there is a localised single tender area known as a trigger spot, which may respond to local anaesthetic injection. As a final resort surgical excision of the tender area may be offered, but in some cases this may make things worse.

BREAST INFECTION

This most commonly affects women of childbearing age and can be divided into those related to lactation and those not related to lactation.

Lactational infection usually occurs during breast-feeding. It presents with pain, swelling and tenderness. The usual organism is staph aureus, and antibiotics should be started (usually flucloxacillin) and the mother should be encouraged to continue breast-feeding to help drain the affected segment. An established abscess may require repeated aspiration or formal incision and drainage.

Nonlactational infection can affect the periareolar region and is often called periductal mastitis. It is associated with smoking, where it is thought that substances in the smoke may damage the breast ducts, which then become inflamed and infected. Treatment is again antibiotics (I&D if necessary to clear a collection). If this fails, care must be taken to exclude an underlying neoplasm. Recurrence is common, since the underlying ducts are damaged and antibiotics do not remove them. If recurrence becomes a problem, then the diseased ducts can be surgically excised.

NIPPLE DISCHARGE

Nipple discharges can be many colours (blood-stained discharges are the most sinister) and can come from either a single duct or multiple ducts. Physiological nipple discharge is common and can range in colour from white to green or black. Other nonmalignant causes of discharge include a duct papilloma or duct ectasia.

A duct papilloma may present with a blood-stained discharge from a single duct and the differential diagnosis includes an underlying carcinoma, which must therefore be excluded.

Mammary duct ectasia (MDE) affects an older age group and presents with a greenish nipple discharge. It is a condition in which there is dilatation of the larger breast ducts, which can also become inflamed and infected. Occasionally this can present with redness and tenderness around the nipple [do not confuse this condition with periductal mastitis (PDM), in which there is inflammation but the ducts are not dilated; patients with PDM are usually younger and there is no association between MDE and smoking]. Any infection associated with MDE may respond to antibiotics, but incision and drainage is not indicated because ductal fistulae can develop. Therefore, if any surgery is contemplated it would be to remove the whole of the affected area.

A careful history should be taken and an examination performed. It is important to note whether a single duct or multiple ducts are involved. The secretion can be sent off for culture and cytology if there is enough of it. Some form of imaging of the breast is necessary in order to exclude an underlying cancer. If all the tests are normal and the discharge is from multiple ducts and not blood-stained, no treatment apart from reassurance is necessary. If the patient remains anxious or the discharge affects her lifestyle, or if a single duct is involved and is persistently blood-stained, then the affected duct can be removed by microdochectomy. In this procedure a probe is passed into the affected duct and the surrounding tissue is excised and sent to histology.

11

LUMPS IN THE HEAD, NECK AND SKIN

Questions on lumps in the head, neck or skin are common in finals, particularly in the short case section of the exam. Students often find these difficult, because they have not prepared separate techniques for examining the different types of lumps. It is easy to forget things under pressure, so you should prepare ways of assessing the common lumps in advance. Do not forget to look and feel inside the mouth and examine facial nerve function when you suspect a parotid lump, and remember to examine draining lymph node groups if there is any chance that a lump could be malignant. Remember also that common things occur commonly and that, as well as lumps specific to the head and neck, lumps such as sebaceous cysts, lipomas, neurofibromas and skin tumours on the head, neck or face are also common short cases in finals.

When any lump is examined you should think of the following list of features:

Site, size, shape, colour, contour (edge), consistency, compressibility (fluctuance), temperature, tenderness, tethering, transilluminance, pulsatility and spread (this means to examine the regional lymph nodes).

This is easy to remember by: SSS, CCCC, TTTT and PS. When describing a lump you do not need to note each of these features — just the ones relevant to the particular lump. For example, a breast lump may be described as "a 3 cm irregular, firm lump in the upper outer quadrant of the left breast, with no associated lymphadenopathy".

LUMPS IN THE HEAD AND NECK

Triangles of the Neck (Figure 11.1)

Conventionally lumps in the neck are described in relation to certain anatomically defined landmarks.

Lumps in the neck anterior to the anterior border of the sternocleidomastoid muscle are within the anterior triangle of the neck (its boundries are the sternocleidomastoid, the midline and the lower border of the mandible). Lumps posterior to the anterior border of the sternomastoid are within the posterior triangle of the neck (boundaries — sternocleidomastoid, trapezius and the clavicle). Lumps under the jaw are in the submandibular region. Therefore, if you are shown a lump in the neck, decide into which triangle it fits and you may almost have the diagnosis already. Remember that lymph nodes can occur in any of the areas (including the parotid) and·can be multiple or single, and that lumps in the midline are invariably thyroid or thyroglossal cysts.

Branchial Cysts

Branchial cysts are relatively rare in practice but are common in examinations. They are believed to represent retained elements of the second branchial cleft which have failed to disappear during embryological development. However, they are not present at birth but appear subsequently, usually in young adult life. They may also be associated with a sinus or a fistula. They are lined by squamous epithelium and are often surrounded by lymphoid tissue. They contain so-called "glary" fluid containing cholesterol crystals. On examination a branchial cyst will usually be a swelling emerging under the anterior border of the sternomastoid muscle at the junction of its upper and middle thirds. If a sinus or a fistula is present, it usually opens at the anterior border of the sternomastoid and the junction of its middle and lower thirds. Treatment is by excision, which may be difficult because the track can extend back to the lateral pharyngeal wall through the fork of the carotid artery.

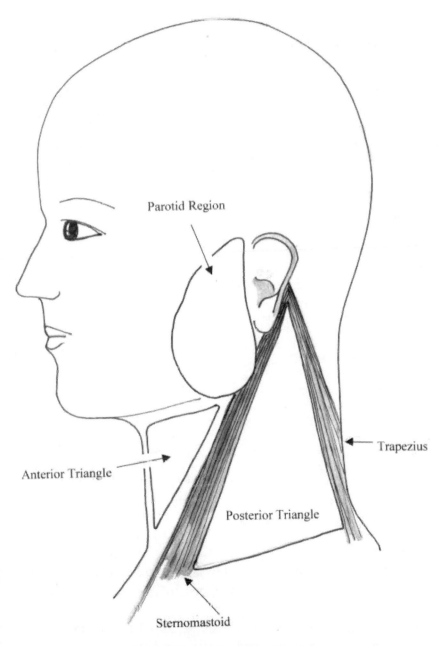

Parotid Region

Trapezius

Anterior Triangle

Posterior Triangle

Sternomastoid

Figure 11.1. The triangles of the neck.

Cystic Hygroma

This is a lump which usually presents in infancy. It is usually found in the lower part of the posterior triangle. It is also known as a cavernous lymphangioma, because histologically it consists of multiple lymph-filled spaces. Clinically it is soft and poorly compressible. It increases in size when the child cries or coughs, and is said to be brilliantly translucent when transilluminated. You are unlikely to see a case in finals, but it is commonly asked about. Treatment is by excision.

Dermoids

These are congenital inclusions found at sites of embryological fusion, such as the angles of the eyes and mouth, and in the midline. They are not common but are often asked about. Treatment is by excision.

Pharyngeal Pouch

(See section on oesophageal disorders.)

Carotid Body Tumours

Carotid body tumours, also called chemodectomas, arise from the cells of the carotid body found at the carotid bifurcation. They usually present as asymptomatic lumps in the neck. Patients are usually middle-aged or elderly. Most of these tumours are benign, although about 10% may metastasize. Clinically they should be suspected when a lump under the sternomastoid muscle has a strongly transmitted pulsation. Investigations include imaging with CT, ultrasound and MRI. On angiography the characteristic appearance is of splaying apart of the carotid bifurcation. Treatment consists of excision by a surgeon used to dealing with the carotid artery.

Thyroid

Lumps in the thyroid are very common in the clinical section of finals, although the management of thyrotoxicosis and myxoedema per se is usually considered under "medicine". In the short cases listen very carefully to what the examiner asks you to do. If asked to "examine the thyroid" you should start with the hands, etc. If asked to "examine the neck" you should just examine the neck and only then do a more general examination of the thyroid, including hands and eyes if you think the lump is in the thyroid gland.

First, inspect the neck from the front, looking for masses. If a mass is seen ascertain if it moves up on swallowing. This is best done by asking the patient to take a mouthful of water. A glass of water next to a patient in finals is often a clue that it is a thyroid patient. If there is not a glass of water, always ask the examiners for one — do not attempt to do the test unless they tell you to. Next, feel the neck. This is usually best done by standing behind the patient, but first check that the trachea is central by placing a finger in the suprasternal notch. From behind palpate the thyroid. If a lump is present decide on its size and whether is it is solitary, multiple or a diffuse enlargement of the whole gland. Again ask the patient to take a mouthful of water and see if the lump moves upwards on swallowing. Now feel for cervical lymphadenopathy and other neck lumps. Then go around to the front again, look into the mouth for any lingual thyroid (at the back of the tongue) and percuss over the sternum for dullness (which may indicate retrosternal extension) and listen for a bruit (present if the thyroid is very vascular). If you suspect thyroid disease, then the hands are inspected for temperature, tremor, pulse rate (tachycardic or AF), and there are five eye signs that go with Graves' disease (exopthalmos, lid retraction, lid lag, opthalmoplegia and chemosis).

If the thyroid feels normal, examine for lymphadenopathy or any other lumps and decide what they are based on the site and characteristics. If you cannot feel any lumps and there are no skin lesions, then check the neck pulses, listen for bruits, and test sensation and neck movements. Bimanual palpation may also be appropriate.

If you are asked to examine "the neck" of a patient, it is perfectly reasonable to examine as above and then say: "This lady has a 4 × 4 cm lump just to the left of the midline that moves upwards on swallowing. This is consistent with a lump in the left lobe of the thyroid gland. The lump is firm, with a smooth contour. I could not feel any other lumps or any associated lymphadenopathy. The trachea is central. There is no retrosternal extension detectable clinically and I could not hear a bruit on auscultation. I would now like to examine this patient for signs of thyroid disease." The examiner will then either tell you to go on or, more likely, ask you what you would look for.

Goitre

The word "goitre" means any swelling of the thyroid gland. The pathology books can make the causes of goitre very complicated, but from a clinical perspective the situation is more straightforward. First, ascertain whether the swelling appears to involve the whole thyroid gland or whether it is a swelling in just part of the thyroid gland. This can be attempted on clinical examination, but in practice nowadays many goitres will require an ultrasound scan to fully decide this. Ultrasound also provides the opportunity for cytology of a solid lesion or aspiration of a cyst.

Causes of Goitre

(A) *Diffusely Swollen Thyroid*
- Hashimoto's thyroiditis (an autoimmune condition)
- De Quervain's thyroiditis (also called subacute thyroiditis — usually a self-limiting condition)
- Iodine deficiency / ingestion of goitrogens (rare)
- Multinodular colloid goitre with nodules too small to detect clinically

(B) *Multiple Nodules in the Gland*
  - Multinodular colloid goitre (the commonest thyroid swelling to be seen in finals)
  - Multiple cysts
  - Multiple adenomas or carcinomas (unusual)

(C) *Solitary Nodule in the Gland*
  - Cyst
  - Tumour (benign or malignant, primary or secondary)
  - Predominant single nodule in multinodular goitre

Multinodular Colloid Goitre

This is thought likely to be an autoimmune condition. It is more common in middle-aged women and there may be a family history. The goitre may be asymptomatic; however, it may be a cosmetic worry to the patient or it may actually be causing symptoms, usually by pressure on adjacent structures, i.e. dysphagia (pressure on the oesophagus) and stridor (pressure on the trachea). In the longer term it may lose its capacity to function, resulting in hypothyroidism. If it is asymptomatic, no intervention is likely to be required other than reassurance and tests to exclude a carcinoma. If it is causing symptoms, then usually a thyroidectomy will be performed. For benign colloid goitre the normal procedure would be a subtotal thyroidectomy, i.e. removal of most of the thyroid but leaving a small amount laterally in relation to the superior thyroid artery to protect the parathyroid glands and recurrent laryngeal nerves and to retain some thyroid tissue to produce thyroxine and prevent hypothyroidism.

Solitary Thyroid Nodules

Ultrasound and clinical examination can determine whether the goitre consists of a single nodule or multiple nodules. However, the mainstay of diagnosis nowadays is by fine needle aspiration for cytology. This is very good at making a diagnosis although it cannot differentiate between follicular adenomas and follicular carcinomas. As discussed above, multiple nodules are usually benign whereas solitary nodules may be malignant. Occasionally a radioisotope scan can be performed to look for a "hot" or "cold" spot. A nodule is said to be "cold" if it fails to take up radioiodine; this is worrying as between 10 and 15% of these nodules are malignant. Radioisotope scanning has less of a role nowadays than it did in the past in the investigation of a thyroid lump.

Fine needle aspiration (if necessary under ultrasound guidance) should be the first line investigation of any thyroid lump. However, if the lump is clincally suspicious then a hemithyroidectomy is usually performed to get a histological diagnosis.

Thyroid Cysts

If large these may present as a lump which may be unsightly or may even cause pressure symptoms. The important thing is to rule out a malignancy. An FNA may be all that is required to show that this is a simple cyst. An ultrasound scan will help if the diagnosis is in doubt. Treatment is by aspiration, but the cyst may require excision if it recurs.

Thyroid Function Tests

Thyroxine (T4) is the hormone produced by the thyroid. It is converted to the active hormone tri-iodothyronine (T3). The thyroid-stimulating hormone, TSH, is produced by the pituitary and stimulates T4 production. There is a negative feedback mechanism in action.

- T3 and T4 are low and TSH is high in hypothyroidism.
- T3 and T4 are high and TSH is low in hyperthyroidism.
- T3 and T4 are normal and TSH is low in patients on adequate doses of T4.

Before any patient with thyroid disease is operated on, it is essential to know the thyroid status by sending off thyroid function tests (TFT's).

Hyperthyroid patients should be controlled as well as possible preoperatively with antithyroid drugs, otherwise they are put on beta-blockers to prevent a thyroid crisis.

Some centres insist on having the vocal cords checked preoperatively to document any abnormalities prior to surgery.

Primary Thyroid Tumours

(i)   *Adenomas.* These are benign and may be either functioning (when they can cause hyperthyroidism and appear "hot" or "warm" on a thyroid isotope scan) or nonfunctioning (when they appear "cold" on a thyroid isotope scan). Treatment is usually by thyroid lobectomy.

(ii) *Follicular carcinoma (25%).* This is found in young adults and is characterised by follicular appearance on histology. It has an extremely good prognosis if appropriately treated. It usually spreads via the vascular system. Treatment is usually by total thyroidectomy. Since the tumour is sensitive to iodine the patient can be given radioiodine to target the metastases (the radioiodine must be administered postoperatively, so that it does not get concentrated in the thyroid gland).

(iii) *Papillary carcinoma (70%).* Like follicular carcinoma, this occurs in younger patients. Spread to lymph nodes is common but does not alter the good prognosis. Treatment is usually by hemithyroidectomy, although some surgeons would perform a total thyroidectomy. Radioiodine is given postoperatively for metastases.

(iv) *Medullary cell carcinoma (5%).* This is a tumour derived from the calcitonin-producing C-cells. It is relatively rare and is part of the MEN-I syndrome. Treatment is by thyroidectomy. It does not take up radioiodine.

(v)   *Anaplastic carcinoma (rare).* This is a highly aggressive and locally invasive tumour and is seen in older patients. It is usually incurable, and treatment is usually palliative but may involve a debulking procedure.

(vi) *Lymphomas.* Lymphomas may also arise within the thyroid gland. They are treated by excision and then standard treatment, depending on the type of lymphoma and stage.

COMPLICATIONS OF THYROID SURGERY

A relatively common question in surgical finals relates to the complications of thyroid surgery or, alternatively, what you would warn someone about who is going to have thyroid surgery. The following should be the basics of such an answer:

(1) *Acute haemorrhage.* Bleeding into the neck after throidectomy can be a life-threatening complication, as it can cause acute airway obstruction. If you are called to a patient in whom this is occurring, the clips or stitches should be removed from the wound and the haematoma evacuated.

(2) The *recurrent laryngeal nerve* runs close to the superior thyroid artery and is at risk during thyroidectomy unless it is specifically identified and preserved. Damage to one recurrent laryngeal nerve causes hoarseness of the voice; damage to both causes airway obstruction requiring tracheostomy (because the neutral position of the vocal cord is in the midline).

(3) *Damage to the parathyroid glands.* This produces hypocalcaemia resulting in tetany. The two physical signs often asked about are Chvostek's sign and Trousseau's sign. Chvostek's sign is when twitching of the facial muscles occurs on tapping over the facial nerve at the posterior aspect of the parotid gland. Trousseau's sign is when carpal spasm is produced by blowing up a blood pressure cuff on the upper arm.

(4) *Hypothryoidism*, due to lack of functioning thyroid tissue.

Thyroglossal Cyst

In embryological development the thyroid starts at the foramen caecum at the back of the tongue and descends to its final position after doing a loop around the hyoid bone. Remnants can be left at any point along this line of descent, including a lingual thyroid (i.e. thyroid tissue at the back of the tongue). Care needs to be taken before excision of a lingual thyroid, in case it is the patient's only functioning thyroid tissue. The classical features of a thyroglossal cyst are that it is in the midline of the neck and rises upwards on protrusion of the tongue. Excision usually involves excision of the central portion of the hyoid bone and may require dissections as far as the back of the tongue. A thyroglossal fistula can also occur, again usually in the midline, but is not actually congenital; it usually occurs following infection or inadequate surgical removal of a thyroglossal cyst.

Parathyroids

The parathyroids only very rarely produce a palpable neck lump (in fact it is so rare that it should probably never be suggested in finals). The management of hyperparathyroidism is, however, a common question.

Most cases of hyperparathyroidism are discovered by finding an elevated calcium on routine investigation. Remember that the symptoms of hypercalcaemia are "bones, stones, psychic moans and abdominal groans" and that hyperparathyroidism can be either of the following:

- *Primary*, i.e. spontaneous (85% due to an adenoma of one gland, 15% due to diffuse hyperplasia of all four glands). In most adenomas parathormone-related protein (PTH-rP) is produced.
- *Secondary*, where hyperparathyroidism is secondary to a low serum calcium such as is found in chronic renal failure and malabsorption syndromes (the PTH is therefore high, with a low or normal serum calcium).
- *Tertiary*, where in long-standing secondary hyperparathyroidism the gland has become autonomous (high PTH and normal or high calcium).

The surgical treatment of hyperparathyroidism is exploration of the neck through a scar similar to that used for thyroidectomy and identification of all four parathyroids. If the cause is an adenoma, it is removed. If it is hyperplasia of all four glands, then three and a half are removed.

Salivary Glands

The salivary glands consist of the parotid, the submandibular, the sublingual and other minor salivary glands.

The parotid region is that part of the face in front of the ear and below the zygomatic arch. The gland is delineated into superficial and deep portions by the branches of the facial nerve. This is why you should examine VII nerve function and also why it is so important clinically to recognise that a lump may be in the parotid gland as simple excision could result in a VII nerve palsy. The operation to remove most superficial lesions of the parotid (superficial parotidectomy) involves making a long incision in front of the ear and down onto the neck, and identifying the facial nerve as it enters the parotid gland. The branches of the facial nerve are then followed forward and the superficial part of the parotid gland dissected off them. If a parotid lump is easily palpable when examined bimanually with a finger in the mouth, it may be in the deep portion of the gland and excision is then associated with a much higher risk of damaging the VII nerve. The facial nerve supplies the muscles of facial expression, so test the nerve by asking the patient to smile, show you his teeth and close his eyes.

Acute Parotitis

In acute parotitis, the gland is surrounded by a tough fibrous capsule, and when it swells, the stretch to the capsule causes severe pain. This condition may be due to viral infection (mumps, coxsackie A and others) or bacterial infection. Bacterial infections usually arise because of obstruction of the duct, usually due to calculus, or because of reduced salivary flow, such as in the postoperative patient or sick dehydrated patient from other causes. This is why mouth care is so important in such patients. Acute bacterial parotitis may result in abscess formation.

Salivary Calculi

Submandibular calculi are the most common type of salivary calculi and may be demonstrated by a plain X-ray or by contrast injection into the salivary duct (called a sialogram). The typical history would be of pain and swelling of the gland in question on eating (due to the production of saliva in an obstructed gland). If the stone is in the submandibular duct in the floor of the mouth, the calculus may be intraorally palpable and easily removed surgically. If it is within the submandibular gland itself, then removal of the whole gland will be required. Parotid calculi are also reasonably common but not usually palpable or easily seen on a plain X-ray. Sialography is usually required to demonstrate them (remember that the duct opens opposite the second upper molar).

Salivary Gland Neoplasms

Salivary neoplasms are common cases in finals. They are usually in the parotid gland (75% of all salivary neoplasms are in the parotid). Most of them are pleiomorphic adenomas.

- *Pleiomorphic adenoma.* This is the commonest salivary neoplasm. It is called pleiomorphic because histologically it appears to be made up of different types of tissue. 90% occur within the parotid. They are slow-growing and benign but the tumours have microprocesses which invade locally and make them prone to recur locally if treated by simple enucleation. They need formal excision by superficial parotidectomy.
- *Adenolymphoma (Warthin's tumour).* This is a benign cystic tumour which contains epithelial lymphoid elements. It occurs in middle

and old age and gives rise to a soft, well-defined cystic lump in the parotid.

* *Adenoid-cystic carcinoma.* This is a highly malignant tumour of the parotid gland. It often causes facial nerve palsies, unlike benign parotid tumours, and is usually hard and fixed on examination. It is often incurable.

SKIN LUMPS

Most of the surgically important skin conditions present as "lumps". You will be expected to be able to examine and describe them and arrive at a reasonable list of differential diagnoses. For many skin lumps, however, the final diagnosis may only be made after excision biopsy, usually under local anaesthetic.

BENIGN LESIONS

Lipomas

These are very common "lumps" in finals. They are benign tumours of adipose tissue. Typically they consist of a soft swelling not fixed to skin or deeper structures. The edge may be difficult to define in some cases and the swelling will often be fluctuant since fat is liquid at body temperature. Dercum's disease is a condition which runs in families where patients have multiple subcutaneous lipomata. Lipomas need removing if they are causing a problem to the patient or are unsightly. Very rarely, a large lipoma can give rise to a liposarcoma.

Neurofibromas

These are benign tumours of nerves which may be multiple and part of von Recklinghausen's neurofibromatosis and associated with café au lait patches. The diagnosis is made by excision biopsy of one of the lesions. They are usually small, firm, smooth, and not fixed to skin or deeper structures.

Sebaceous Cysts

These follow obstruction to the mouth of a sebaceous duct. They are common on the scalp but can occur anywhere except the soles and the palms (which do not have sebaceous glands). Typically they form a round, soft swelling attached to the skin but not deeper structures. A central punctum may be visible and usually clinches the diagnosis. Sebaceous cysts contain cheesy material which may become infected. Less commonly, they may ulcerate or form a sebaceous horn. They are usually simply removed under local anaesthetic.

Benign Naevi (Pigmented Moles)

Surgically the main importance of benign naevi is in the differential diagnosis of malignant skin lesions, principally malignant melanoma.

Papillomas

Papillomas arise from either squamous or basal layers of the skin. They include:

- Infective warts — due to viral infection.
- Keratin horns.
- Basal cell (seborrhoeic or senile) warts. These occur in elderly patients and are often multiple and may be pigmented.
- Pedunculated papillomas (skin tags). These are of no medical significance but may need removing if they are catching on clothes or are a worry cosmetically.

Campbell de Morgan Spots

These red spots appear as patients grow older and are of no clinical significance. They need no treatment.

MALIGNANT LESIONS

Melanomas

The incidence of malignant melanoma is rising sharply. Exposure to ultraviolet radiation is thought to be the major aetiological factor (especially sunburn as a child).

Melanomas are highly malignant tumours derived from melanocytes and need to be diagnosed and removed early if a cure is to be produced. Fair or red-haired individuals are at the highest risk. The commonest sites are the torso in males and the legs in females (suggesting that sun exposure is a risk factor). Rare sites include the nail bed (acral lentiginous), the anorectal junction and the choroid in the eye. If you come across a patient in the exam with a glass eye and an enlarged liver, think melanoma!

Any mole which either grows or appears rapidly, changes shape or colour, itches, ulcerates or bleeds should be regarded as suspicious and removed.

The types include:

- Superficial spreading melanomas (about 80%) — these grow slowly and metastasise late, and have a better prognosis.
- Nodular melanomas — these invade deeply and metastasise early, and have a poorer prognosis.

Total excisional biopsy is the method of choice for diagnosis, although in some circumstances (for example in a huge lesion) a partial biopsy is necessary.

You need to be familiar with two staging systems used for melanomas. The *Breslow thickness* is the depth of the tumour in millimetres and gives a good indication of the prognosis. Another system is *Clark's staging*, which breaks down the depth into five anatomical levels (e.g. Stage I — confined to the epidermis; and Stage V — penetrated into the subcutaneous fat). In practice the two are combined together with the histological grade to give a more accurate stage.

Prognosis

The thickness of the primary tumour is the single most important prognostic factor for patients with no evidence of distant spread.

As a rough guide the following table lists the five-year survival rates based on the depth:

Thickness	Five-Year Survival (%)
< 0.76 mm	96–99
0.76–1.50	87–94
1.51–4.0	66–77
> 4.0	< 50

Tumours in the BANS areas (back, arms, neck and scalp) tend to do worse than tumours on the periphery. Women seem to survive longer than men, and this may be due in part to their having more tumours on the legs than men. Various histological types (such as those with increased mitoses) and those with satellite lesions (implying that the dermal lymphatics are involved) have a worse prognosis. Ulceration is a poor prognostic indicator.

The surgical margins for resection are still controversial but, as a rough guide, impalpable lesions (thought to be < 1 mm) should have a 1 cm margin whereas thicker palpable lesions (> 1.5 mm) should have a 2–3 cm clearance. Survival is independent of the width of excision, but local recurrence may not be. Dissection of the regional lymph nodes is again a controversial subject, but most surgeons would agree that this should only be performed if they are clinically palpable.

Other modalities used include chemotherapy and isolated limb perfusion, although with limited success and prognosis is not greatly improved. Close follow-up of out-patients is important in order to detect recurrence early.

Basal Cell Carcinomas

Basal cell carcinomas (BCC's) are very common lesions and are often asked about in finals or seen as short cases. They are low grade malignancies, rarely metastasising, but they can erode into bone or other adjacent structures if they are left to grow large enough. Exposure to sunlight is a risk factor but they do not occur until middle age or later. 90% are found on the face, usually above a line from the lobe of the ear to the corner of the mouth. Early lesions consist of a raised pearly pink papule with fine telangectasia over it. Later the lesion ulcerates and is often called a "rodent ulcer". Treatment is usually by surgical excision, although cryotherapy or radiotherapy is sometimes used.

Squamous Cell Carcinomas

Squamous cell carcinomas (SCC's) are less common than basal cell carcinomas, but once again exposure to sunlight is a risk factor. With these and BCC's a cumulative effect of UV light appears to be important, whereas with melanomas short periods of intense exposure (burns) appear to be responsible. SCC's are more malignant than BCC's and may arise in pre-existing lesions such as leg ulcers (when they are called Marjolin's ulcers). Metastasis is often to regional lymph nodes, which should always be examined. Treatment is by excision, with radiotherapy being used to treat recurrence or involved lymph nodes.

Bowen's Disease

This is characterised by single or multiple brownish plaques, usually well defined and slightly raised and scaly. It is an intraepidermal squamous carcinoma.

Kaposi's Sarcoma

This tumour is increasingly seen because of its association with HIV. It usually consists of raised purplish nodules which may be single or multiple.

12

HERNIAS

Hernias are common cases in surgical finals and are also often asked about in the written papers. Their assessment is usually straightforward if a common sense approach to their examination and management has been developed and practised.

DEFINITIONS

A fairly common question is to ask you to define a hernia. We would suggest the use of the following definition:

A hernia is the protrusion of a viscus or part of a viscus through the walls of its containing cavity into an abnormal position.

When writing an answer on hernias, remember that they can also occur in sites away from the abdomen, such as when there is herniation of the brain through the foramen magnum with raised intracranial pressure or herniation of a muscle through a fascial defect in the leg. These other types of hernia should be mentioned for a complete written answer, although they should certainly not be more than a small part of any general answer about hernias. In the clinical section of the exam, however, you are very unlikely to see anything other than abdominal hernias. Abdominal hernias may be external (i.e. they emerge to the subcutaneous tissues as with inguinal hernias — so there is a lump to feel) or internal (such as with hiatus hernias, where there is no lump to feel).

There are a number of terms applied to (abdominal) hernias and it is worth defining these:

- *Sac.* The sac is the peritoneal lining of the hernia. Within it are the contents of the hernia (usually intestine or omentum). The sac may be complete or incomplete (i.e. not surround all the contents), as is found in a sliding hernia.
- *Neck.* The neck of a hernia is the margin of the defect through which the hernia has emerged.
- *Reducible.* A hernia is reducible when its contents can return to the abdominal cavity either spontaneously or with manipulation.
- *Irreducible.* The hernia cannot be reduced despite pressure or manipulation.
- *Incarcerated.* This term is usually used to describe an irreducible hernia where the irreducibility is due to adhesions within the sac in the absence of obstruction or strangulation. Some textbooks, however, define it as meaning a hernia which is irreducible because of faeces within the large bowel. Perhaps because of this confusion about the true definition of this term, it is best simply to refer to a hernia as being irreducible but not obstructed or strangulated.
- *Obstructed.* The bowel within the hernia is obstructed. The patient may have the four cardinal signs of obstruction (pain, vomiting, distention and constipation).
- *Strangulated.* The blood supply to the contents of the hernia is occluded by pressure at the neck of the hernia. If the bowel is within the sac, the viability of the bowel is impaired. Usually the veins are occluded first and then further swelling leads to arterial occlusion, which precedes gangrene developing. If the hernia contains only omentum, then this too can strangulate, but in this case bowel obstruction does not occur.
- *Sliding hernia.* A sliding hernia is one which contains a partially extraperitoneal structure, such as the caecum on the right or the sigmoid colon on the left. Therefore, the sac does not completely surround all the contents of the hernia. The importance of this is that particular care must be taken when excising the sac, to avoid damaging the bowel.
- *Richter's hernia* (see Figure 12.1). This is where just part of the bowel wall is caught in the sac, and may become strangulated.

Because only part of the bowel wall is in the sac, the patient is not usually obstructed.

- *Herniotomy.* This term is used to describe ligation and excision of the hernia sac.
- *Herniorrhaphy.* This term is used for actual repair of the hernia defect.

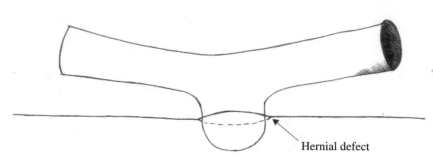

Figure 12.1. Richter's hernia.

The natural progression of a groin hernia could therefore be that the patient notices a lump in the groin that is reducible, and this may go on for years. Then, one day, the lump becomes irreducible, implying that it had become incarcerated. The patient may be well at this point. The lump may then become painful and the overlying skin reddened, implying strangulation (he may or may not have symptoms of obstruction, depending on whether there is bowel within it). At this point this becomes a surgical emergency and the patient requires an urgent operation to relieve the ischaemia.

CLASSIFICATION OF HERNIAS

Hernias require a defect in the wall of their normal cavity for their formation. This defect may be of two types:

- Congenital
- Acquired

Congenital

The commonest types of congenital hernias are inguinal and umbilical hernias appearing in childhood.

Infantile inguinal hernias are usually seen in males. In males, when the testes develop and descend *in utero* they pass down and through the abdominal wall into the scrotum, forming what will subsequently develop into the inguinal canal. As this happens a finger-like projection of peritoneum, called the processus vaginalis, is carried down with the testicle. This usually obliterates, but if it remains patent fluid or abdominal contents may enter down it, forming either a hydrocoele (fluid around the testicle) or a hernia (containing bowel or omentum). The treatment is simple operative ligation of the processus vaginalis, i.e. a herniotomy.

Umbilical hernias are commonly seen in infants and represent failure of complete obliteration of the umbilical opening. They often disappear spontaneously and rarely strangulate. Surgical repair should therefore be reserved for those which persist after the age of five and those with a defect greater than 1 cm in size.

Acquired

To acquire a hernia, a weakness of the abdominal wall has to be produced. The following may be predisposing factors:

- Chronic cough
- Chronic constipation (and straining to pass faeces)
- Straining to void urine (prostatism)
- Severe muscular effort (heavy lifting)
- Obesity
- Weakening with age
- Surgery

GROIN HERNIAS

Groin hernias are the commonest type of hernia encountered in finals, and indeed they account for about 75% of all hernias. They may be

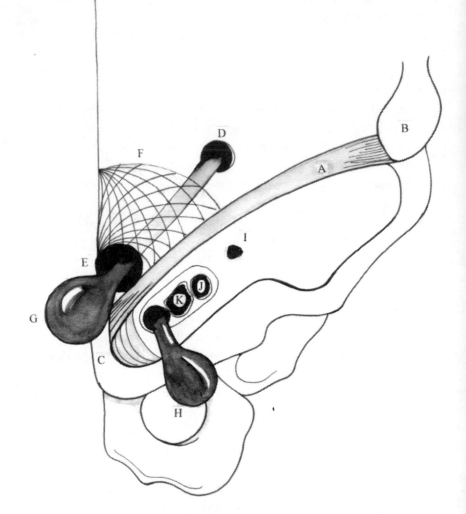

Figure 12.2. Anatomy of the groin. (A) Inguinal ligament inserting onto pubic tubercle, (B) anterior superior iliac spine (ASIS), (C) symphysis pubis, (D) deep inguinal ring, (E) superficial inguinal ring, (F) external oblique aponeurosis, (G) indirect inguinal hernia, (H) femoral hernia, (I) femoral nerve (outside femoral sheath), (J) femoral artery, (K) femoral vein.

either femoral or inguinal. Inguinal hernias are further divided into direct and indirect. Inguinal hernias are proportionally more common in males than in females, and femoral hernias are proportionally more common in females than in males (possibly because of a wider pelvis and hence femoral canal). In both sexes, however, inguinal hernias are more common than femoral hernias in absolute numbers. Hernias may present in three ways:

(1) As a lump (which may come and go; classically the lump would appear on straining or lifting and disappear on lying down or when pressed on by the patient).
(2) With pain in the groin.
(3) Because of a complication (obstruction or strangulation).

To understand groin hernias properly some basic anatomical knowledge is required.

Femoral Hernias

Femoral hernias emerge through the femoral canal, which normally contains only fat and lymph nodes. The medial border of the femoral ring (the upper and widest part of the femoral canal) is the sharp-edged lacunar ligament, which makes these hernias more prone to strangulation than inguinal hernias. Anteriorly is the inguinal ligament, posteriorly is the pectineal ligament and laterally is the femoral vein. Consideration of the position of the femoral canal will show why these hernias emerge below and lateral to the pubic tubercle. If identified all femoral hernias should be repaired because of the risk of strangulation. Elective repair involves excision of the sac (herniotomy) and repair (herniorrhaphy), usually by suturing the inguinal ligament to the pectineal ligament with interrupted nonabsorbable sutures. Emergency repair is similar but usually utilises an incision through the inguinal canal or abdominal wall so that the bowel can be carefully assessed for strangulation and a bowel resection performed if necessary.

Inguinal Hernias

Inguinal hernias emerge into the subcutaneous tissues through the superficial inguinal ring and thus emerge above and medial to the pubic tubercle (see Figure 12.2). They have, however, left the abdominal cavity above and lateral to the pubic tubercle to enter the inguinal canal. This point often confuses finals students, especially as in a thin patient a cough impulse or hernia bulge can be seen or palpated above and lateral to the pubic tubercle beneath the external oblique aponeurosis (i.e. it is within the inguinal canal and has not yet emerged from the superficial inguinal ring).

Inguinal hernias are classified into direct and indirect. Indirect hernias leave the abdominal cavity through the deep inguinal ring along with the structures of the spermatic cord. Some of these may be due to a patent processus vaginalis (see "infantile hernias" above) which has not presented until adult life. Direct inguinal hernias enter the inguinal canal "directly" through a weakness or defect in its posterior wall. Both then emerge through the superficial inguinal ring. Indirect hernias, because of their close association with the spermatic cord, often then extend down into the scrotum. Direct hernias rarely extend into the scrotum.

Students are often asked in exams to assess whether a groin hernia is inguinal or femoral. The key to this is the position of the pubic tubercle in relation to the point where the hernia emerges into the subcutaneous tissues. A hernia emerging above and medial to the pubic tubercle is an inguinal hernia, whereas a hernia emerging below and lateral is a femoral hernia. Sometimes a hernia is so large that it may appear anywhere in relation to the pubic tubercle. In this case the key is to reduce the hernia, place your finger on the pubic tubercle and ask the patient to cough and see where the lump emerges from.

Once a diagnosis of an inguinal hernia is made, students may be asked to comment as to whether they feel the hernia is direct or indirect. To our mind this is largely an unfair and pointless exercise, since good studies have shown that even consultant surgeons are often wrong when it comes to this assessment; the only way to be certain is to see which it is at the operation, and anyway it does not alter the surgical approach. However, if asked you must be able to carry out the relevant assessment with skill and confidence. Your confidence can legitimately be increased by the knowledge that your examiner may not be able to get the correct answer himself. The basis of the test is to reduce the hernia, then apply pressure with a finger over the deep inguinal ring. The patient should then be asked to cough or strain. If the hernia is controlled it is probably indirect, but if it comes out anyway it may be a direct hernia (most of those we say are direct are in fact indirect).

Of some controversy is the actual site of the deep inguinal ring. Most surgical textbooks state that it is about 1.5 cm above the mid-point of the inguinal ligament, which is slightly lateral to the mid-inguinal point (the site of the femoral artery). However, most anatomy textbooks suggest that the deep inguinal ring is directly above the mid-inguinal point (i.e. above the femoral pulse), in which case the mid-point of the inguinal ligament becomes redundant as a landmark!

The treatment of an inguinal hernia consists of excision of the sac (herniotomy) and repair of the posterior wall of the inguinal canal and deep inguinal ring (herniorrhaphy). The older operations involve suturing the posterior wall of the inguinal canal with nonabsorbable sutures, but repairs are now being introduced where a nylon mesh is used to close the defect, producing less tension in the sutures and therefore less pain and a lower risk of sutures cutting out leading to a recurrence of the hernia. Such nylon meshes can be inserted either at open operation or by a laparoscopic technique.

Differential Diagnosis of a Lump in the Groin

Occasionally a lump in the groin will be something other than a hernia. The list of differential diagnoses includes:

- Inguinal lymph nodes (often multiple and usually below the inguinal ligament)
- Saphena varix, a dilated varicose vein at the sapheno-femoral junction (disappears on lying flat, and there may be other varicosities in the legs)

- Femoral artery aneurysm (pulsatile)
- Encysted hydrocoele of the cord (can get above it)
- Lipoma of the cord
- An incompletely descended testicle (absence of the testicle on that side)

Remember you cannot get above a hernia and these other lumps will also not usually exhibit the classical features of hernia:

(1) Cough impulse
(2) Reducibility
(3) Bowel sounds heard over the hernia

Although a single enlarged femoral node can sometimes be difficult to distinguish from a strangulated femoral hernia containing omentum, such cases will rarely be seen in finals. Usually, if care is taken to examine the patient lying down and standing, the diagnosis will become obvious. Remember also to carefully examine both groins (as hernias are often bilateral) and the scrotum as there may be associated epididymal cysts or hydrocoeles to find. This is particularly important for the short case section of the exam, where questions such as "This patient has a lump in his groin — examine him and tell us what you think" are fairly common.

Here is a summary of how to examine "a lump in the groin":

(1) Introduce yourself and ask the patient if he minds your examining him.
(2) Expose the abdomen, groin and legs. Ask the patient to stand, and inspect for any obvious lumps or scars and comment on your findings (if the patient is already lying it is perfectly reasonable to perform the examination in this position; however, you must stand him at the end of the examination, or you may miss small hernias, saphena varices and varicocoeles.
(3) Examine the genitalia and both groins. If you can see an obvious lump feel it gently and ascertain the features of the lump. Ask the patient to cough and feel for a cough impulse, listen over it for bowel sounds, and ask him if he is able to reduce it.

Once it is reduced find the pubic tubercle and place your index finger on it. Ask the patient to cough and observe where the lump appears from in relation to your finger. An inguinal hernia will come out from the inguinal canal above and medial to your finger, whereas a femoral hernia will protrude below and lateral.

If you think this is an inguinal hernia, then state, for example, "The patient has a 5 cm smooth lump in his right groin. I think this is an inguinal hernia, because I cannot get above it, it is reducible, exhibits a cough reflex and protrudes above and medial to the pubic tubercle." The examiner might then ask you to tell if it is direct or indirect.

(4) If a scrotal swelling is present determine if it has an upper border, remembering that you cannot get above a hernia. Therefore, a lump with no upper border is likely to be an inguinoscrotal hernia. If you can get above it, then it is likely to be either a cord or a testicular lump. Ask yourself two questions: Is it separate from the testis, and does it transilluminate? Do not forget to feel the epididymis and the skin of the scrotum as well (see Figure 14.1).

Other Types of Hernia

Incisional Hernias

These can be simply defined as hernias which arise through a previously made incision. They are often broad-necked and, therefore, have a low risk of strangulation. Factors leading to the development of an incisional hernia include obesity, old age, chronic cough or straining due to constipation or prostatism (i.e. things which increase intra-abdominal pressure), postoperative wound infection or haematoma and poor surgical technique when the wound is closed. In high risk patients even large incisional hernias are often managed conservatively with an abdominal elastic support corset. Repair may be difficult and require the insertion of a nylon mesh to allow closure of the defect without tension.

Umbilical Hernia

In adults the hernia usually emerges adjacent to the umbilicus (unlike the congenital type) and is usually termed "paraumbilical".

Richter's Hernia

This is a hernia where only part of the circumference of the bowel is within the sac. It is most often seen with femoral hernias. This is the only type of hernia which can strangulate without obstructing (other than hernia which contains only the omentum). Although rather unusual in practice, it seems remarkably common in exam questions, which is why you need to know about it (see Figure 12.1).

Epigastric Hernia

This hernia arises in the mid-line through the linea alba. It is usually small and often difficult to feel, especially in overweight patients. It rarely contains bowel but often has extraperitoneal fat. It can cause symptoms out of proportion to its size, however, and patients often undergo unnecessary investigations for other causes of upper abdominal pain before the correct diagnosis is eventually made.

Spigelian Hernia

Again this is very rare but common in exam questions. It is a hernia which occurs into the posterior rectus sheath at the point where the posterior sheath becomes deficient (i.e. at the arcuate line of Douglas).

Obturator Hernia

This hernia occurs into the obturator foramen and does not usually produce a palpable lump. It is most commonly seen in thin elderly women, and pressure on the obturator nerve gives rise to pain felt on the inner aspect of the thigh. It is usually diagnosed only when obstruction has occurred, often not being suspected prior to laparotomy. The typical presentation would be a thin old lady with distention, vomiting, colicky abdominal pain, absolute constipation and pain in the inner thigh.

13

VASCULAR DISEASE

INTRODUCTION

Vascular patients constitute a significant minority of the cases seen in surgical finals, and in addition many written papers will have some questions about vascular surgery. Most cases will be covered within the categories of arterial disease or venous disease, and most patients with venous disease will have varicose veins or venous leg ulcers. Questions about deep venous thrombosis and pulmonary embolism are usually considered part of general medicine. The exception relates to prophylaxis against DVT for surgical patients — this is a very common question. Questions relating to cardiac surgery are not usually considered fair game for surgical finals except in their relation to cardiology, which again comes under general medicine.

Unfortunately many students have not been given the opportunity to work in a vascular unit or vascular firm and they often find this a confusing area when it comes to preparation for the finals. As vascular surgery is a fairly specialised area, students will not be expected to know anything about the minutiae of the specialty. What would be required, however, is a good knowledge of the principles of the following areas:

(1) How to examine the vascular system
(2) Management of the acutely ischaemic leg
(3) Management of the chronically ischaemic leg
(4) Management of aneurysms
(5) Management of carotid artery stenosis

In addition, make sure you know how to feel the pulses, including the popliteal, dorsalis pedis and posterior tibial pulses, and do not forget to listen for bruits. Also remember the importance of identifying risk factors such as smoking, diabetes and hyperlipidaemia.

ARTERIAL DISEASE

Examination of the Peripheral Arterial System

Examination of the peripheral arterial system should obviously be included as part of a full cardiovascular examination and as part of a full examination of a patient in the long case section of the finals. However, it may be helpful to detail how one would carry out an examination restricted to the peripheral arterial system.

First of all, one would inspect the patient for signs of peripheral arterial disease, such as ulcers, gangrenous toes, previous amputations, peripheral cyanosis, etc. In order to do this the patient must be adequately exposed, and usually the examination will be done with the patient supine, with no clothes on except for something to cover the genitalia to preserve his dignity. Do not forget to look for abnormal pulsations that might be caused by abdominal aortic aneurysm. The examination then proceeds with inspection of the hands and feeling of the radial pulses. These should be felt individually on both sides and the two sides then compared. Likewise the brachial pulses should then be felt and compared. The brachial pulse is best palpated just above the elbow crease on the medial aspect of the upper arm. A surprising number of patients have radial pulses which are difficult to feel, whereas the brachial pulse is usually highly palpable unless there is an arterial occlusion higher up. If there is doubt about the pulses being present or being equal, then it would be appropriate to suggest taking the blood pressure in each arm in order to get a more objective confirmation of this. There should not be more than 15 mm of mercury difference between the blood pressure in the arms unless there is a vascular problem.

The next part of the peripheral arterial examination is checking of the carotid pulses. Remember that the common carotid, which divides into the internal and the external carotid, is within the carotid sheath which lies under the anterior edge of the sternocleidomastoid muscle. The best way to feel the carotid pulse is with the patient's head resting on one pillow; ask him to look to the opposite direction, and then feel under the sternocleidomastoid. It is then important to listen for a bruit over the carotid. The best way to do this is to ask the patient to take a breath and then hold it whilst you listen with the diaphragm of the stethoscope. If you listen whilst he is breathing, you will find it difficult to hear soft bruits because of the noise made by the air moving in and out of the trachea. The process is then repeated for the carotid on the other side of the neck. Do not palpate the two carotids at the same time, as some patients may faint if that is done. If you are examining the cardiovascular system in general, then it would be appropriate at this point to move on to examination of the heart; if not, the next step is to examine the abdomen.

First of all, look for pulsation which might be caused by an aortic aneurysm, and then palpate for such an aneurysm. Then the abdomen should be auscultated for bruits. Remember that a bruit heard in the upper abdomen may be due to renal artery stenosis. Remember also that the bifurcation of the aorta is at the level of the umbilicus and so aneurysms are usually felt in the upper abdomen.

The next stage of the arterial examination is to check the pulses in the groins and legs. The femoral pulse should be palpated on both sides and one side compared with the other. In coarctation of the aorta there may be radiofemoral delay. This is manifested by feeling the radial and femoral pulses simultaneously and feeling that the femoral pulse wave is occurring fractionally after the radial pulse. Coarctation of the aorta is, however, very uncommon. Such patients are usually young and often present with severe hypertension, so do not be tempted to overdiagnose this condition.

After palpation of the femoral artery, noting also whether it is of normal calibre or aneurysmal, auscultation of the femoral artery should be carried out to listen for bruits.

The next thing to do is to feel for the popliteal arteries. This should be done routinely, as otherwise one may miss a popliteal aneurysm. It is, however, often very difficult to feel the popliteal arteries in many patients, especially if they are overweight. Indeed, it is said that if one feels the popliteal pulse very easily one should suspect immediately that there is a popliteal aneurysm present. There is no shame therefore for any student who says he cannot feel the popliteal arteries, but it is important that you do know how to examine them properly, and this is one area of examination of the peripheral arterial system that many students fall down on badly, perhaps because doctors who are not vascular surgeons either miss out the examination of the popliteal arteries or do it badly themselves. The best way to proceed is as follows:

The patient's leg should be almost straight and you should take great care to try and get him to relax the leg as much as possible. The principle of the method for feeling the popliteal arteries relates to fact that there is a triangular bare area on the lower end of the femur between the heads of the gastrocnemius muscle and it is against this bare area that one tries to press up into the popliteal fossa so that the pulsation can be felt between the fingers and the bone. To do this, one needs to have a counterpressure, and this is done by resting the thumbs on the front of the knee and then gently pushing up into the popliteal fossa with the first and second fingers of both hands at the same time.

The next part of the peripheral arterial examination is to feel the foot pulses. There are two pulses which are normally palpated: the dorsalis pedis pulse (which is absent in 10% of normal people) and the posterior tibial pulse. The dorsalis pedis pulse is found on the dorsum of the foot in the groove between the extensor tendons of the big toe and the second toe. The posterior tibial pulse is around about a centimetre behind the medial malleolus, just above the level of the ankle joint. Again these pulses can be difficult to feel and there is no shame in saying that you could not feel them. You must, however, look professional in the way you palpate them, and of course feeling for them in the wrong position looks very bad indeed. The commonest fault that students make when trying to feel the foot pulse is in fact to press too hard. This results in your being much more aware of the pulse in your own fingers as well as making the pulse in the artery more difficult to palpate. Whilst you are examining the foot pulses it would be appropriate to just look again at the foot in more detail than was done at the start of the examination. The foot should be felt to see whether it is warm, and the two sides compared. Any pallor or cyanosis should be commented on, as well as any areas of ulceration or necrosis. It is often useful to test for capillary return and compare the two sides. This is normally done by pressing on the pulp of one of the toes for a second or two to make it blanch and then seeing how long it takes for the colour to return. Unfortunately this test may be influenced by the patient having cold peripheries or being generally shut down, but a difference between the two sides is suggestive of arterial disease.

The final clinical test which you need to know about is something called Buerger's test. This is done by elevating the legs to an angle of about 50°. Ideally the two legs should be elevated at the same time. They should be kept up for about 2–3 min and the rate at which the skin blanches should be observed. Again differences between the two sides are often more useful than any absolute change. After this period of elevation the legs are swung over the edge of the bed and put into a dependent position (ideally the patient is placed in a standing position). You should then look for the rate at which the veins in the foot refill, again comparing the two sides. Then look at the rate at which colour returns to the leg. If the blood supply is poor, then after about 2 min the foot develops an intense hyperaemic response called reactive hyperaemia. This is due to vasodilation caused by the accumulation of products of anaerobic metabolism during the period of elevation. In practice you may not be required to actually do this test in the examination, but you may be asked about it and you should certainly know the principle of the test.

Management of the Acutely Ischaemic Leg

Patients with an acutely ischaemic leg will not be found in the clinical cases section of final exams, but it is a relatively common question in vivas and in written papers as to how one would identify and manage a patient with an acutely ischaemic leg.

A useful way to remember the clinical signs and symptoms is the so-called list of 6 P's:

Pain, Pallor, Pulselessness, Parasthesiae, Paralysis and Perishing cold

Of these paralysis and parasthesiae are the two which indicate severe ischaemia threatening the loss of the limb. Remember also that the two commonest causes of acute ischaemia of the leg are an embolus and a thrombosis.

Embolism most commonly comes from the heart, where a thrombus has formed because of atrial fibrillation, heart valve disease or myocardial infarction. More rarely, emboli may be thrown off into the arterial circulation from aneurysms of the thoracic or abdominal aorta. Although it occurs extremely rarely, most students seem to have heard of the so-called *paradoxical embolus*, where a DVT thrombus passes into the arterial circulation through a septal defect of the heart, thereby getting into the arterial circulation instead of causing a pulmonary embolus as it would usually do. Although this is incredibly rare, it is one of those interesting little facts which seem to pepper finals and which therefore you probably need to know about.

Thrombosis is the other main cause of acute ischaemia and usually occurs on top of pre-existing arterial disease. In such patients there may thus be a history of pre-existing claudication and pulses may be absent in the opposite leg as well as in the symptomatic one.

Because of the relatively poor ability of muscle and nerve cells to cope with prolonged ischaemia, acute leg ischaemia needs to be treated as a surgical emergency and revascularisation should be produced within 4–6 h if the limb is to be saved.

An embolus is suggested by the absence of any previous vascular history (i.e. claudication), the presence of normal pulses in the other leg and the presence of atrial fibrillation. There is some debate as to exactly what sequence of events should be preferred, but most surgeons would agree that if it is clearly an embolus then the patient should be taken without delay to theatre for an emergency embolectomy. This is done by exposing the femoral arteries in the groin. The arteries are then opened after clamps have been applied and a special catheter, called a Fogarty balloon embolectomy catheter, which is basically a long thin flexible catheter with a balloon on the end, is passed down the artery with the balloon deflated. Once it has been passed as far as possible the balloon is gently blown up and the catheter is drawn back, pulling out any thromboembolus with it. This catheter was designed by Thomas Fogarty when he was a medical student, and questions about it seem to come up fairly often in surgical finals.

Once the thomboembolus has been removed, the arteriotomy (i.e. incision in the artery) can be closed and the procedure is over. A sample of the embolus is usually sent for histology as well as culture. This is to exclude two of the rarer causes of peripheral emboli, namely an atrial myxoma (a benign tumour arising in the atrium of the heart) and an infected thrombus forming in subacute bacterial endocarditis. The patient should then be started on heparin whilst investigations to identify the source of the embolus are carried out, such as echocardiography.

If a thrombosis is suspected rather than an embolus, then it is usually best to try and arrange for the patient to have an arteriogram carried out before going to theatre, as an embolectomy will probably not be sufficient. Arteriograms can be performed either by injection of contrast material into the venous circulation with films being taken as the contrast subsequently passes into the arterial circulation, or by direct injection into the arterial circulation. The commonest site for the injection for peripheral arteriography is through the femoral artery, when a catheter is then passed up into the aorta before contrast is injected. Many hospitals have facilities to do a procedure called digital subtraction angiography, in which a computer system is used to subtract the images from before and after injection of the contrast so that structures such as the bones and soft tissues are removed, thereby improving the resolution of the image of the arteries. Depending on the precise findings of the angiogram, the leg will often require some form of bypass surgery in order to restore blood flow (as in chronic ischaemia). After successful restoration of flow it is usual to divide the deep fascia of the calf (i.e. a "fasciotomy") to prevent damage occurring if the muscles swell. Care must also be taken to avoid renal failure caused by myoglobin leaking out from damaged or dead muscle (i.e. "myoglobinuria"). These are termed reperfusion injuries.

Management of the Chronically Ischaemic Leg

Minor degrees of narrowing of major arteries may be completely asymptomatic. As narrowings progress or as occlusions occur, the degree of symptoms will depend on the anatomical level of the occlusion or stenosis as well as the presence of collateral vessels. For most patients with peripheral vascular disease, the first thing they will notice is pain in the calf muscles when they walk, so-called vascular claudication, and this is due to muscle ischaemia. The pain then disappears on resting. The only condition which commonly mimics this is pain due to lumbar spinal canal stenosis, so-called spinal claudication. In these patients, however, rather than true pain they usually suffer with numbness and pins and needles when they exercise and the symptoms are not usually well localised to the calf muscles as they are with true vascular claudication. As the degree of arterial occlusion worsens, the patient may suffer shorter and shorter distance claudication before eventually getting rest. Unlike the calf pain of claudication, rest pain is usually felt in the foot or toes (rest pain is ischaemia of muscles and also the soft tissues at rest). This typically occurs at night and the usual history is that the patient wakes due to the pain and has to hang the foot out of bed or walk on a cold floor in order to gain some relief. The reason the pain occurs at night is that we lose the effect of gravity helping to supply blood to the feet, and also that the cardiac output drops when we are asleep and the warmth of the bedclothes causes vasodilation to the skin diverting the blood from the soft tissues.

Patients who have severe arterial disease sufficient to give them rest pain are usually classified as having something termed "critical ischaemia". Critical ischaemia can be loosely defined as ischaemia which is severe enough to threaten the loss of the limb or part of the limb. It can also be defined with the help of something called the "ankle brachial index". Basically this involves taking the blood pressure in the foot using a blood pressure cuff on the calf and a Doppler probe in order to pick up the foot pulse signal in either the posterior tibial or the dorsalis pedis pulse. The cuff is blown up until the signal disappears, and this is taken as the systolic pressure in the foot. This systolic pressure is then taken in a similar way in the arm, and the ratio of the two is calculated. The normal ankle brachial index (ABPI) is 1 or slightly greater than 1. In claudication it is usually between 0.5 and 0.9. Below 0.5 the patient may start to suffer with rest pain or, if more severe, perhaps necrosis or gangrene of the toes. Occasionally a claudicant may have a normal ABPI at rest, but this will be found to drop on exercise when an increased blood requirement to the muscles is limited by the stenosis.

Currently most vascular surgeons would agree that patients with mild claudication are best managed conservatively, with the main advice being "stop smoking and keep walking". In addition medical problems such as anaemia, hypertension, hyperlipidaemia, diabetes and heart failure should be corrected. Overweight patients should be advised to lose weight.

For more severe claudication or where there is thought to be a high chance of an iliac artery lesion, an angiogram should be arranged to see if there is an angioplastiable lesion. Treatment of patients with chronic arterial disease may be carried out either by radiological intervention, i.e. balloon angioplasty, or by surgery. Balloon angioplasty consists in passing a special catheter into the narrowed area of the artery in a way similar to that in which an angiogram is carried out. The balloon on the end of the catheter can then be blown up to a high pressure to stretch open the narrowing. Angioplasty is a good technique in that it does not involve an anaesthetic and can be done with relatively little risk to the patient. It is particularly useful for narrowings or short occlusions of the iliac arteries but is less good for disease below the inguinal ligament. Usually, only when there is either critical ischaemia or severe claudication which is making the patient's life intolerable should surgery be considered. In general terms there are only a small number of vascular surgical procedures which are commonly carried out and specific details will not be required for surgical finals. Occlusion in the aorta or iliac artery is usually treated by an aorta-bifemoral bypass graft, in which an artificial graft, usually made of Dacron, is taken from the aorta above the blockage down to the femoral arteries in the groin. In patients who are considered too unwell to undergo this fairly major procedure, the femoral arteries can be revascularised by taking a graft from the axillary arteries just beneath the clavicle and running this down the sides of the thorax and abdomen under the skin into the groin arteries. In a patient with one good femoral pulse but a blocked iliac artery on the opposite side, a similar result can be achieved by taking a graft from the good common femoral artery across the subcutaneous tissue suprapubically into the ischaemic leg. This is termed a "cross-over graft".

For blockages further down the leg either a femoral-popliteal or a femoral-distal procedure may be performed ("distal" in this context means "distal to the popliteal artery", i.e. to one of the three tibial vessels — posterior tibial, anterior tibial and common peroneal). The preferred choice of graft for these bypasses is usually the long saphenous vein, which may be either used with its valves destroyed by a special valve-cutting instrument or reversed so that the valves do not interfere with blood flow. Only if a suitable vein is not available do vascular surgeons resort to using an artificial graft material for grafts below the inguinal ligament. The commonest artificial material used below the inguinal ligament is polytetrafluraethylene (PTFE).

In broad terms, the further down the leg the graft goes the less likely it is to work, such that for femoral distal bypasses only about 50% of them are still working at one year.

Aneurysms

The word "aneurysm" comes from the Greek word for "widening" and is usually applied to abnormal widening of the arteries. Aneurysms can be found at various sites within the arterial circulation (e.g. aortic, femoral and politeal). Berry aneurysms are found within the arteries in the circle of Willis and, if they rupture, can cause subarachnoid haemorrhage. These are not usually considered under general surgery, but aneurysms of the peripheral arterial system are.

Causes of Aneurysms

Most aneurysms are so-called atherosclerotic aneurysms. This means that they appear to be caused by atherosclerosis and the patients have the risk factors for this. Other, rarer causes of aneurysms include connective tissue disorders such as Marfan's syndrome and Ehlers–Danlos syndrome. Another, relatively uncommon cause of aneurysms is syphilis. Although rarely seen nowadays, it used to be a common cause of aneurysm.

Atherosclerotic aneurysms share some of the risk factors for ordinary peripheral arterial occlusive disease, such as smoking and hypertension. However, there is probably an underlying genetic tendency, as these aneurysms also appear to run in families. They are more common in men and are rarely found before the age of 50 years, suggesting that there may also be an underlying predisposition to form aneurysms on top of specific precipitating risk factors.

Complications of Aneurysms

There are a number of possible complications for all aneurysms:

(i)   Rupture
(ii) Thrombosis
(iii) Distal embolisation
(iv) Pressure on adjacent structures
(v)   Fistula into adjacent structures such as vena cava or intestine
(vi) Infection of the aneurysm thrombus

These complications can all occur to a greater or lesser degree, with arterial aneurysms at different sites.

Abdominal Aortic Aneurysms

Aneurysms of the abdominal aorta affect the segment of aorta below the renal arteries in 90% of cases. Aneurysms that go higher than the renal arteries usually require an incision through both the chest and the abdomen for their repair. These are called "thoracoabdominal" aneurysms. Whilst nowadays infrarenal aortic aneurysms should have an elective mortality rate of less than 10%, ruptured abdominal aortic aneurysms have a mortality rate of approximately 50%.

The best screening test for abdominal aneurysms is an ultrasound scan, which is cheap and provides a reliable method of sizing the aneurysm. In patients where surgery is to be considered or where the exact level of the aneurysm in relation to the renal arteries is in doubt, further imaging including a CT scan or an MRI scan may be needed. An important point to remember is that most abdominal aortic aneurysms are lined with a thick layer of organised thrombus. This means that the lumen size of the aneurysm is very much smaller that its overall size. An angiogram will therefore not show the true extent of the aneurysm, as it only outlines the lumen of the vessel. Hence angiograms are not of great help in assessing aortic aneurysms and are usually done only in those patients who also have symptoms suggestive of occlusive arterial disease. Likewise, angiograms are not useful in following up cases where the mainstay is usually still the ultrasound scan.

Infrarenal abdominal aortic aneurysms of less than 5 cm in maximum diameter are usually managed conservatively. The question is: When do you decide to operate? The crucial factors that come into this decision are the risk of rupture, the operative mortality, and the age and general condition of the patient. Therefore, if the risk of rupture is considered to be much greater than the risk of the opertion, then surgery is sensible. Aneurysms of greater than 6 cm maximum diameter will usually be recommended to have surgery if the patient is fit enough. Aneurysms between 5 and 6 cm, however, present a more difficult problem, as precise rupture rates are not known and the question of surgery should be decided principally in relation to the patient's general fitness. Key points in assessing fitness for surgery include an assessment of cardiac, respiratory or renal problems. Of these, cardiac disease is the most common cause of mortality following aneurysm repair and should be assessed carefully with a full history, focusing specific attention on getting details of the patient's exercise tolerance.

As mentioned above, aortic aneurysms of greater than 5 cm in size will normally be operated on if the patient is considered fit enough. Symptoms such as abdominal or back pain or tenderness when the aneurysm is palpated are thought to represent an increased risk of rupture, and such patients are usually also recommended to undergo urgent surgery. Ruptured aneurysms should of course be taken immediately to theatre, with no delay in investigation or resuscitation. Effectively these patients will not survive unless "the tap is turned off".

Surgery is traditionally by "open" operation where the upper end of the aneurysm, called the "neck of the aneurysm", is clamped below the renal arteries and then an artificial graft is sewn inside the aneurysm sac either down to the bifurcation of the aorta, i.e. using a straight graft, or onto each iliac artery, i.e. using a bifurcated graft. The graft material often used is Dacron. Nowadays some aneurysms are repaired using less invasive radiological techniques, although currently these are available only in a small number of highly specialised centres.

Popliteal Aneurysms

Popliteal aneurysms are found less commonly than abdominal aortic aneurysms, although 50% of patients with a popliteal aneurysm will also have a coexistent aortic aneurysm. A popliteal aneurysm should be suspected when the popliteal pulse is unusually prominent or easily palpated. Whilst with abdominal aortic aneurysms the major risk is rupture, popliteal aneurysms seem to rupture rarely and the most common complication is acute thrombosis of the aneurysm causing acute ischaemia. Such an event usually requires emergency surgery with femoropopliteal bypass grafting. If it is identified before thrombosis has occurred, then grafting and tying-off of the aneurysm should be carried out electively in order to prevent the catastrophe occurring.

Aneurysms at other sites are relatively unusual. Those that involve the thoracic aorta obviously require extremely major surgery for their repair, with attendant high rates of morbidity and mortality. Aneurysms of the visceral arteries, such as the renal arteries or splenic arteries, have a tendency to present only after rupture, and also have a relatively high rate of mortality because of this.

It is very unlikely that a student will be asked to see cases other than infrarenal or popliteal aneurysms in surgical finals. One thing to be aware of, however, is the case where there is ectatic (i.e. tortuous) arteries which may feel aneurysmal when palpated from the outside. The commonest situation where this occurs is in the carotid arteries, where an ectatic carotid artery may easily be mistaken for a carotid artery aneurysm. Another situation to be aware of is where a mass lying in front of an artery (such as a pancreatic cancer in front of the abdominal aorta) is felt as a pulsatile mass. This pulsation is, however, transmitted only to the mass. The key to diagnosing a true aneurysm is to demonstrate expansile pulsation whereby the mass can be shown to be truly expanding in size with each pulse when examined using both hands.

CAROTID DISEASE

Typically, atherosclerosis of the carotid arteries occurs at the point where the common carotid divides into the internal and external carotid arteries. Narrowing or occlusion of the external carotid artery does not usually matter clinically because of the rich collateral arterial network within the head and neck. Stenosis or occlusion of the internal carotid artery is, however, potentially much more serious and can cause either strokes or transient ischaemic attacks. The precise details of the neurology related to these events should be sought in medical textbooks. However, in summary, a transient ischaemic attack is described as a neurological deficit which completely reverses within 24 h of its onset. A stroke is obviously a neurological deficit which persists for longer than 24 h. Amaurosis fugax is an ischaemic event usually due to an embolus passing through the retinal arterial circulation and is effectively a type of transient ischaemic attack ("amaurosis fugax" simply means "fleeting blindness" in Latin).

Clinically, carotid artery stenosis may be diagnosed either because of a finding of a bruit over the carotid artery on examination or, after investigation, because of a transient ischaemic attack or a stroke. The main investigation used to screen for carotid artery stenosis is duplex ultrasound scanning of the carotid artery. In addition angiography may be used to confirm the severity and type of stenosis. There is now good evidence (from two large multicentred trials that took place in the US and in Europe) that symptomatic carotid stenosis of greater than 70% should be treated by carotid endarterectomy in patients who are otherwise well. If these patients are treated with medical therapy only (i.e. aspirin), they have a significantly increased risk of stroke. The operation of carotid endarterectomy involves incision over the anterior border of the sternocleidomastoid muscle in the neck and dissection of the common, internal and external carotid arteries. The common and internal carotid arteries are then opened using a longitudinal incision at the site of the stenosis, and the atheroma is "cored out" and the artery closed. In some patients it may be necessary to put in a temporary plastic bypass tube in order to maintain blood flow to the brain during this operation. The major complication of the procedure is a perioperative stroke (at the best centres this risk is 5% or less).

When a carotid stenosis has been found in an otherwise asymptomatic patient, the role of surgery is much less clear, and this is currently the subject of clinical trials.

VENOUS DISEASE

Varicose Veins

Medical students often find varicose veins a rather daunting case to meet in surgical finals, because they have not prepared a systematic way of examining them and presenting their findings. This is a mistake! At least one varicose vein patient is to be found in most surgical short case exams. These patients are plentiful on most hospital waiting lists and they are usually quite happy to come up to participate in finals, with the offer of getting their operation done rather more quickly than it might be otherwise. Usually the patients who have been selected will have quite obvious and significant varicose veins, and at first sight examination can be daunting in view of the large number of varicosities that they may have.

Probably the best way to consider how to approach a case of varicose veins is first to consider how varicose veins arise. Simplistically, we can think of the deep venous circulation as being at a higher pressure than the superficial venous system. Where the two systems join there are valves which have the purpose of preventing the pressure within the deep system coming out into the superficial system. If these valves go wrong (i.e. become incompetent), then the superficial veins dilate up and appear as varicose veins. The common sites where this may occur in the lower limb are firstly at the long saphenous femoral vein junction in the groin (this is the commonest site), secondly at the short saphenous popliteal vein junction in the popliteal fossa behind the knee, and thirdly from so-called perforating veins (veins which pass directly from superficial to deep) which become incompetent. Calf perforating veins are usually found on the medial side of the calf. Typically there are three: one just above the medial malleolus, one a hand's breadth higher and one hand's breadth higher than that. In addition some patients have a perforator in their medial thigh which is usually connected to the long saphenous vein. The position of perforators may, however, vary.

When one is assessing a patient with varicose veins, it is therefore important to try and categorize the varicose veins into three groups:

(a) Long saphenous veins
(b) Short saphenous vein
(c) Veins arising from calf perforators

In addition the patient may have disease of the deep veins which may either be obstructed or incompetent, or may have a leg ulcer.

Points in the History

It is important to ascertain what it is about the varicose veins that troubles the patient. He may just be worried about them from a cosmetic point of view. Alternatively, he may be getting aching pains which are usually worse after a period of standing. Some patients find that they get swelling of the ankles, again most often after a period of standing. Varicose veins do sometimes cause cramps and other nonspecific pains in the leg, but one must always be on the look-out for other pathology which might be causing the pain, as many patients will immediately ascribe pain from any cause (arthritis of the knee, for example) to their obvious and visible varicose veins.

Other points in the history which are usually taken include asking for a family history of varicose veins, any previous medical history suggestive of deep venous thrombosis or pulmonary embolism and, most important, whether the patient, who is usually a young woman, is on the oral contraceptive pill as this is something that really should be stopped six to eight weeks before surgery because of the risk of DVT. Most varicose veins in women seem to worsen after pregnancy, and it is also a good idea to enquire about the number of past pregnancies and whether the woman wishes to have further pregnancies in the future. Some surgeons will suggest delaying treatment if that is the case.

Points on Examination

Never forget that occasionally abdominal or pelvic masses (including pregnancy) or malignancies can present as varicose veins due to pressure on the inferior vena cava or iliac veins. A full examination of the abdomen should therefore be part of examining a patient for varicose veins. In the short case section of the final examination, you may not be expected to do this by the examiner (because of a lack of time), but you should make a point of mentioning that "I would now wish to do a full abdominal examination".

Another point not to forget is to examine the arterial pulses in the legs. This is especially important in patients who have a leg ulcer.

Varicose veins will usually be best seen with the patient standing up. The legs should be exposed from the groin to the toe. As with all clinical examinations, the inspection should come first. You should particularly be looking for the presence of any signs of current or past leg ulceration. In patients who have had long-standing varicose veins and venous hypertension, you may see the changes of skin pigmentation (the skin is

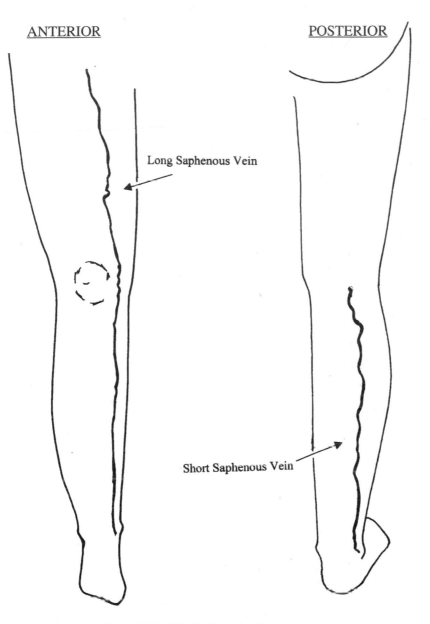

Figure 13.1. Distribution of varicose veins.

brown in colour, due to haemosiderin deposits) or lipodermatosclerosis (there is atrophy and loss of elasticity of the skin and subcutaneous tissues). Because most patients with significant skin changes will have calf perforator disease, and because the calf perforators are found on the medial side of the calf above the medial malleolus, these changes are usually most prominent in the medial lower calf. In addition you should inspect the veins to try and make some preliminary judgment as to whether it seems they are likely to be arising from the long saphenous, short saphenous or perforating system. Remember that the long saphenous vein runs from the groin down the medial aspect of the thigh and calf. The veins below the knee which arise from it will therefore be mostly situated on the medial side of the calf, and in a thinner patient you may see a dilated varicose long saphenous vein running up the thigh. The short saphenous veins arise from the popliteal vein at a variable level within the popliteal fossa and then runs down to the lateral side of the calf. By just looking at the legs with the patient standing you may be able to make a good guess as to which of these two patterns the veins fall within. Calf perforating veins, which are incompetent, may produce very few varicosities but, as mentioned earlier, they will often be associated with significant skin changes of pigmentation and lipodermatosclerosis. Therefore, one can usually make a preliminary (educated) guess as to which of the three categories the veins fall into just on inspection.

Next comes palpation. Patients with a prominent saphena varix at the saphenofemoral junction may actually have a lump visible in the groin, and this will need to be palpated to make sure it is not due to a lymph node or hernia. Otherwise the mainstay of palpation is the so-called "tap" test, whereby the veins are tapped down on the calf and palpation over the saphenous vein in the thigh will reveal a transmitted thrill if the veins are in continuity. It is also at the stage of palpation that one should quickly check the femoral, foot and popliteal pulses.

Next comes the so-called "tourniquet" test, or Trendelenberg's test. Perhaps it is this which confuses more medical students than any other aspect of varicose vein examination. This test can be adapted to be as complex or as simple as one would wish. In the days before vascular laboratory tests were widely available and reliable, some surgeons used variations of this test involving more than one tourniquet placed at several levels. This is now rarely done. The principle of the test is that it is possible to compress the superficial veins by a tourniquet applied around the leg. The best way to proceed with the test in finals is to get the patient to lie down, and elevate the leg and then milk the veins with your hand to emptiness before applying a tourniquet initially as high on the thigh as possible. Most finals will have available suitable tourniquets. The ones used for taking blood from the arm may not be large enough for some patients' legs. The patient is then asked to stand and the veins are inspected to see if they refill rapidly. Remember that all varicose veins will refill slowly as blood passes through the arterial circulation, through the capillary bed and back into the venous system. What one is looking for is a rapid refilling within a few seconds, indicating that the tourniquet has not prevented the superficial reflux. For example, if there is saphenofemoral junction reflux causing varicose veins, a high thigh tourniquet will prevent this rapidly refilling as the patient stands. If, however, there is short saphenous or calf perforator incompetence, the veins will fill rapidly despite a high thigh tourniquet. If the veins are controlled by the tourniquet in the thigh, then they are long saphenous veins due to saphenofemoral reflux. If they are not controlled, the next manoeuvre should be to position the tourniquet just below the knee and repeat the test. If the veins are now prevented from refilling rapidly, then there is either saphenopopliteal reflux or, very occasionally, a thigh perforator that is incompetent. If the veins continue to fill rapidly despite this tourniquet just below the knee, there is almost certainly calf perforator incompetence. Some people do this test using pressure from the fingers instead of a tourniquet. However, adequate pressure is much more difficult to achieve using this technique, and we would not advise it in finals.

In practice this is the limit to which the tourniquet test can be taken in finals. To expect a student to apply the tourniquet at more than these positions is almost unheard of, and in many cases the examiner will be satisfied with simply describing what you would do and not require you to actually do it. Remember also that some patients will have a mixture of the three types of veins, i.e. long saphenous incompetence and calf or perforator incompetence. In such patients the tourniquet test will be difficult to interpret with any certainty.

Leg Ulceration

Ulceration can have many causes, although by far the commonest is venous disease, which accounts for about 80% of ulcers. The following is a list to help you remember the other causes:

(1) Arterial — due to either major-vessel disease or small-vessel disease, e.g. vasculitis, rheumatoid arthritis.
(2) Neuropathic — most traumatic ulcers have a neuropathic element, e.g. alcoholism, peripheral neuropathy, diabetes, tabes dorsalis and syringomyelia.
(3) Traumatic.
(4) Systemic disease — e.g. pyoderma gangrenosum.
(5) Neoplastic.

Venous ulceration may be either superficial venous incompetence or incompetence of the valves of the deep veins. Venous ulceration will usually be found above the medial malleolous in the position where the calf perforators arise. There will usually be the signs of pigmentation and lipodermatosclerosis. About 10% of leg ulceration is caused by arterial disease. These ulcers may be situated anywhere in the leg or foot and may be associated with other signs of peripheral ischaemia, such as gangrenous toes. 5–10% of patients may have a mixture of the two causing their leg ulceration (this is why you must always feel the pulses). The main differential diagnosis is a neuropathic ulcer. Such ulcers are probably due to repetitive trauma to an area, with absent or decreased sensation. When you are assessing an ulcer, therefore, it is important to decide whether it is a vascular problem (major or small vessel) or whether it is neuropathic. A neuropathic ulcer is painless, the surrounding skin is insensitive and the rest of the foot should be warm, with a good blood supply.

Treatment of Leg Ulceration

Once the cause of the leg ulceration has been investigated, initial treatment may be directed towards underlying causative factors, such as arterial ischaemia, vasculitis, etc. However, the majority of leg ulcers are due to venous disease; it is the management of this which is most likely to be asked about in surgical finals and which the student needs to know in some detail.

The principles underlying treatment for leg ulceration can be summarised as being:

- Dressing of the ulcer
- Pressure bandaging
- Elevation

Systemic antibiotics should be reserved for patients who have a cellulitis surrounding the ulcer. Ulcers are always affected to some degree by colonising skin organisms, and antibiotic treatment does nothing for the rate of ulcer healing and may just breed resistant organisms. A very dirty or sloughy ulcer may require treatment with antiseptic or desloughing dressings initially, i.c. dressings which may contain agents such as iodine or streptokinase. Such agents may, however, impair the rate of epithelial regrowth of an ulcer. After the ulcer becomes clean, simple dressings which maintain a moist environment over the ulcer should be used in order promote epithelial regrowth. Elastic bandaging or graduated compression stockings (these have a higher pressure at the ankle than they do higher in the leg) should also be applied and in addition the patient should be asked to elevate his leg as much as possible. The use of compression bandaging and elevation is to reduce venous hypertension. In severe cases it may be necessary to admit the patient to hospital for elevation and bed rest in order to promote ulcer healing. In some cases where there is a large ulcer with a clean granulating bed, it may be appropriate to consider the use of skin grafting in order to reduce the length of time required for the ulcer to heal.

Finally, an assessment of the venous system should be made, and if there is significant superficial venous incompetence (i.e. long saphenous, short saphenous or calf perforating veins), then consideration should be given to treating this surgically. Unfortunately, when deep venous valve incompetence is present (usually following previous deep venous thrombosis), there is currently no good surgical procedure to improve deep venous function. For such patients the mainstay of treatment is to try and get the ulcer healed using the above methods and then to maintain healing by fitting a good quality elastic graduated compression stocking. Patients who have their ulcers successfully healed should be encouraged to wear such stockings on a life-long basis.

DEEP VENOUS THROMBOSIS AND PULMONARY EMBOLISM

Management of deep venous thrombosis and pulmonary embolism is usually considered part of the medical finals. However, pulmonary embolism is the commonest preventable cause of death in surgical patients, and it is appropriate to be asked about it in surgical exams, especially in relation to prophylaxis.

At an early stage the only signs of a deep venous thrombosis (DVT) may be an increase in warmth and dilatation of the superficial veins. As the thrombosis progresses the leg will swell. At a later stage the leg may be extremely swollen, with impairment of skin circulation (phlegmasia caerulea dolens or phlegmasia alba dolens), and occasionally this may lead to venous gangrene. Pulmonary embolism may present in different ways. Massive pulmonary embolism will produce cardiorespiratory arrest and may initially be misdiagnosed as a primary cardiac problem. A pulmonary embolism should always be suspected in a patient suffering a collapse or cardiac arrest within the first two weeks of their surgical procedure. Less major degrees of pulmonary embolisation may produce lesser degrees of collapse, or perhaps dyspnoea or pleuritic chest pain.

The treatment of deep venous thrombosis is anticoagulation, usually with heparin at first, followed by warfarin. If a patient continues to have pulmonary emboli despite adequate anticoagulation, then he should be considered for insertion of a venocaval umbrella filter.

Prophylaxis Against DVT in Surgical Patients

Patients having anything other than minor surgery should have prophylaxis against deep venous thrombosis. This is particularly so if they have any risk factors, such as age, obesity, cigarette smoking, the contraceptive pill or a previous history of DVT or PE. The commonest type of prophylaxis employed is subcutaneous heparin, usually given two or three times a day (5000 units subcutaneously). It is also common practice to use TED stockings (thromboembolic deterrent stockings), and many units have intermittent pneumatic compression devices which work by blowing up a series of cuffs on the leg and keeping the venous pump flowing even when the patient is immobile or in theatre.

Lymphoedema

This is an abnormal collection of interstitial lymph fluid either due to a congential absence of the lymphatics (primary) or secondary to blockage of the lymphatics.

Primary lymphoedema can be present at birth (congenital lymphoedema), but more often it presents in the teens as lymphoedema praecox (Milroy's syndrome). This usually affects young females who present with progressive swelling (nonpitting) of one or both legs. Less often, it can present late at around the age of 30–40 and is then called lymphoedema tarda.

Secondary lymphoedema can be caused by anything that damages or obstructs the lymphatics. The term FIIT is helpful in remembering the causes:

Fibrosis — e.g. following radiotherapy.
Infiltration — e.g. by tumour, especially prostatic in men and lymphoma in women (in certain parts of the world infestation with filariasis is a common cause for lymphoedema).
Infection — e.g. TB.
Traumatic — e.g. after block dissection of lymphatics.

Treatment of lymphoedema is usually nonoperative. This involves elevation and external compression stockings, and early intervention if infection develops. There are now lymphoedema nurses who use various compression devices, and massage techniques that are very good at reducing the swelling in such patients.

There are no curative surgical procedures available and only the most severe cases come to surgery, which usually involves debulking procedures to improve mobility.

14

UROLOGY

Questions on urology feature quite often in essays and short answers, such as "Discuss the investigations for painless haematuria" or "Discuss the management of benign prostatic hypertrophy". There will be a high chance that you will get a urological problem as a long case, since such patients are usually not too ill before or after their operation to assist with the exams. If you have never seen an irrigation bag and three-way catheter before, you may be caught out. In the short case section you may see a lump in the scrotum, but urology does not feature high on clinical signs.

CATHETERS AND CATHETERIZATION

The most common catheter is the Foley catheter (named after Fredrick Foley in the 1930's). Such catheters have inflatable balloons at the bladder end to hold them in position. They can be two-way (one lumen for the urine and one to allow the balloon to be blown up) or three-way (with an extra lumen to allow irrigation fluid to be passed into the bladder). The balloon can be inflated by injecting about 10 ml of saline, although the newer catheters have a second balloon, filled with saline, built in at the outflow end of the catheter, which when squeezed inflates the other balloon at the bladder end (saving the need for a syringe!). Catheters can be made from different materials, such as latex, plastic or silicone (silastic or long term indwelling catheters). The *external circumference* of the catheter (in millimetres) is sized by the Charriere (Ch), also called the French (Fr) gauge system (to calculate the diameter, divide by π!). Fr 10 is small and Fr 22 is very large. The usual size used for males is size Fr 14 or 16. The catheters have standard lengths, the male ones being about twice as long as the female ones.

Male Urethral Catheterization

Retract the foreskin if the penis is not circumcised, use the aseptic technique (clean the area with antiseptic, one hand holding the penis and the other holding the cotton wool with forceps, and the region is draped), instil anaesthetic gel into the urethra, and introduce the catheter fully into the urethra (the penis is usually held vertically or at 45°); once urine drains, inflate the balloon and connect the catheter to either a free drainage bag or an hourly measuring urine bag. Never inflate the balloon unless you are sure you are in the bladder. Return the foreskin to prevent a paraphimosis. Note the residual volume of the urine and send the specimen of urine for bacteriology. The complications of urethral catheterization include local trauma, introduction of infection, urethritis and stricture formation.

Some centres advocate the need for routine antibiotic cover for this procedure (usually one dose of gentamycin 80 mg IM); others feel this is unnecessary. In certain situations antibiotics are essential, for example if the patient had a metal prosthesis such as a hip replacement or if the patient had a heart murmur, since infection in these patients could be disastrous.

Suprapubic Catheters

Suprapubic catheters are used when urethral catheterization is not possible (e.g. urethral stricture) or is inappropriate, such as when urethral trauma is suspected (pelvic injury with a high-riding prostate). There are many types of suprapubic catheters, and they can either be specially manufactured suprapubic catheters or using a newer special introducer such as the Add-a-Cath; a normal Foley catheter can be used. The Add-a-Cath has a plastic sheath around a sharp-ended trocar. The catheter is inserted into the bladder in the mid-line about 5 cm above the symphysis pubis. The plastic sheath around the introducer can be zipped down and torn off to allow the whole sheath to be removed once the catheter is in the bladder. The only way to understand this properly is to ask a urologist to show you the actual catheter.

Haematuria

Haematuria can be a finding on urine analysis (microscopic haematuria), or the patient complains of passing red urine (macroscopic or frank haematuria). 20% of patients with frank haematuria have a urological malignancy.

Haematuria can be due to general or localized causes. The general causes include bleeding disorders, leukaemias, the use of anticoagulants, haemoglobinopathies and sickle cell disease. The local causes can be bleeding anywhere along the urinary tract — the kidneys, ureters, bladder, prostate or urethra. At any of these sites the bleeding may be due to infections (TB, schistosomiasis or UTI), stones, trauma, tumours, etc. Renal diseases such as glomerulonephritis also cause haematuria.

In your history you should elicit the following points:

(1) Is the blood definitely in the urine and not from the vagina or rectum?
(2) Is it true haematuria? There are many other causes of red urine, including drugs (rifampicin, nitrofurantoin), foods such as beetroot, and systemic disease such as porphyrias or rhabdomyolysis.
(3) Is the haematuria associated with loin pain or pain on passing urine? Pain usually implies stones or infections, whereas painless haematuria should set alarm bells ringing for more sinister causes.
(4) The nature of the bleeding — is it microscopic or macroscopic? Are there any clots in it? Is the bleeding at the beginning of the stream in an otherwise clear stream (suggestive of a urethral or prostatic lesion) or is it throughout the stream (suggestive of a lesion in the bladder, ureters or kidneys)? Bleeding at only the end of the stream is unusual.

Examination of such patients should include an assessment of their general health. Look for signs of anaemia, feel for a renal mass and conduct a digital rectal examination to assess the prostate.

Investigations

(1) *Urine tests.* A mid-stream urine should be dipsticked, and sent for microscopy and culture. The urine should also be sent off for cytological analysis.

(2) *Haematological tests.* Send a full blood count to see if the patient is anaemic, and carry out U & E's to assess renal function.

(3) *Radiological tests.* A plain abdominal X-ray which includes the region of the kidneys, ureters and bladder (known as a KUB) is taken (a normal plain abdominal radiograph cuts out part of the bladder). The soft tissue of the renal tract is not seen well on a plain film, so an intravenous urogram (IVU) is performed, where images of the kidneys, ureters and bladder are obtained after the patient has been given an injection of a contrast medium that is excreted by the kidneys. This is particularly good for looking at the kidneys and ureters, but not so good for looking at lesions in the bladder. An ultrasound of the renal tract can detect tumours in the renal parenchyma and bladder lesions. If a renal mass is seen, then a CT scan is performed.

(4) *Special investigations.* Cystoscopy means a look inside the bladder. This is usually performed under local anaesthesia using a flexible (fibre-optic) cystoscope, but sometimes rigid cystoscopy is needed (for example when the haematuria persists at the time of the cystoscopy and rigid cystoscopy allows a washout to be performed). Other special investigations include early morning urine samples (EMU's) for TB culture and, very rarely, angiography to exclude arteriovenous malformations.

For macroscopic haematuria and persistent microscopic haematuria, an IVU and cystoscopy should always be performed. If these are normal, then an ultrasound scan can be requested.

If given an essay on this subject you should talk about the above and obviously discuss the causes in detail using an aetiological and pathological sieve.

BLADDER OUTFLOW OBSTRUCTION

Bladder outflow obstruction (BOO) is most commonly caused by benign prostatic hypertrophy (BPH) or prostate cancer. Only these two causes will be discussed in detail.

Other causes include bladder neck obstruction (which affects young to middle-aged men and is due to bladder neck dysfunction, treated by bladder neck incision or drugs) and urethral stricture (which is due to urethral trauma, catheterisation, previous transurethral surgery or sexually transmitted diseases such as gonorrhoea, and is treated by urethrotomy and dilators). Bladder calculi can sometimes cause BOO.

Lower urinary tract symptoms can be divided into obstructive and irritative symptoms:

Obstructive Symptoms

- Hesitancy (as a higher bladder pressure is needed to initiate micturition to overcome the obstruction)
- Poor stream
- Intermittent flow and terminal dribbling
- Incomplete emptying [feeling like you need to go again straight away (*pis en deux*), also associated with bladder diverticulae]

Irritative Symptoms

- Frequency
- Urgency (and urge incontinence)
- Nocturia (needing to get up more than once at night)

The aetiology of the irritative symptoms is poorly understood. These symptoms may be secondary to BPH but can also be a feature of intravesical pathology, such as bladder cancer, urinary infections and stones.

The complications of BOO include urinary tract infection as a result of urinary stasis, formation of bladder calculi, hydronephrosis, and acute (painful) and chronic (painless) urinary retention.

BENIGN PROSTATIC HYPERTROPHY (BPH)

The prostate is a capsulated fibromuscular gland, which measures $4 \times 3 \times 2$ cm and normally weighs about 15 g. As the male gets older the gland enlarges, especially in the transitional zone (in contrast to cancer, which affects the peripheral part of the gland). The symptoms are those listed under BOO.

The abdomen should be examined to exclude urinary retention. On *rectal examination* the normal prostate has a smooth surface and there is a palpable mid-line sulcus. In BPH the normal findings are present but the gland is enlarged. The size and consistency should be noted.

Investigations

- Urine should be dipsticked and sent for microscopy and culture. Send U&E's to assess renal function. Prostate specific antigen (PSA) is a protein produced by prostatic acinar cells (both normal and cancerous, although cancerous cells produce about ten times as much). The level of PSA in the blood increases as the prostate increases in size (both BPH and cancer). The PSA also increases with age. The normal PSA is < 4. If the PSA is > 10 the risk of cancer is more likely (however, it can be raised markedly with BPH). A PSA between 4 and 10 is difficult to interpret, and the higher it is the more likely it is to be cancer. If the PSA is high or clinically the prostate is suspicious, then a transrectal ultrasound and biopsy of the prostate can be performed.

- A urine flow test is performed. This involves passing urine onto a flow meter and generates a graph of urinary volume (ml) against time (s). An ultrasound of the urinary tract is usually performed to assess the residual bladder volume and to look for upper tract dilatation, which may result if the obstruction is severe.
- More invasive investigations might include a cystoscopy if a urethral stricture or bladder calculus is suspected or if irritative symptoms predominate. Urodynamic (bladder pressure) studies can be performed for complex cases.
- A voiding diary is helpful in seeing how much bother the symptoms cause the patient.

Management

If the symptoms are mild and do not bother the patient, then a policy of watchful waiting may be adopted, with a review in the clinic to see if the symptoms have changed. Approximately 65% of patients will either not improve or get worse.

As long as there is no evidence of complications of bladder outflow obstruction, such as hydronephrosis, recurrent UTI's or urinary retention, treatment is a choice between surgical and medical options, depending on symptom severity and patient preference.

Medical treatment involves the use of $\alpha 1$ adrenoreceptor blockers such as Indoramin and Terazosin, which relax the prostatic smooth muscle increasing urinary flow, and help with the obstructive symptoms although these can cause postural hypotension. $5\text{-}\alpha\text{-reductase}$ inhibitors such as Finasteride (which block the conversion of testosterone to the more active dihydotestosterone, the hormone important in developing BPH) have been used but are of doubtful efficacy.

Surgical treatment involves removing the obstructing part of the prostate.

Transurethral resection of the prostate (TURP) is the most frequently performed operation for this condition [and the second most common operation (after cataract surgery) performed on men over 60]. The patient is placed in a lithotomy position and a resectoscope, passed through the urethra, is used under direct vision to remove the prostate piece by piece using cutting diathermy, the chippings being sent to histology. Diathermy is also used to stop any bleeding. A three-way catheter is inserted postoperatively to irrigate the bladder until the fluid is no longer heavily blood-stained. This stops any clots forming and blocking the catheter.

Complications of TURP include:
General and specific, early and late, etc.

Early — septic shock, bleeding and transurethral syndrome.

Transurethral (TUR) syndrome is uncommon and is like water intoxication, thought to be due to absorption of hypotonic irrigation fluids during the TUR (saline cannot be used, because it limits the use of diathermy). The problems include electrolyte imbalances (especially hyponatraemia), haemolysis, fluid overload, and if brain oedema occurs the patient can become confused and can fit and lose consciousness. Treatment is difficult but essentially involves fluid restriction, diuretics and close observation.

Late — secondary haemorrhage, urethral strictures, impotence, recurrent prostatic regrowth and recurrent symptoms.

It is essential, when consenting the patient, that he knows that between 65 and 85% will develop retrograde ejaculation (sperm flows into the bladder on orgasm and hence he becomes infertile). Some urologists believe that impotence might occur in up to 3–5% of patients postoperatively, although this is debatable.

TURP is the gold standard treatment of BPH. As so many men develop BPH, a day case procedure is being sought which will be as effective as TURP. Newer methods for treating BPH include microwave therapy, laser prostatectomy, radiofrequency ablation and prostatic stents (find out which technique is used at your hospital). Open prostatectomy (retropubic or transvesical) is only performed nowadays for very large prostates where the gland is larger than 100 g and TURP would take too long, leading to a high risk of TUR syndrome developing.

UROLOGICAL CANCERS

Carcinoma of the Prostate

The symptoms are usually those of benign prostatic hypertrophy and it is therefore difficult to differentiate between carcinoma of the prostate (CaP) and BPH. CaP can be diagnosed histologically after TURP for what was thought to be benign disease when the prostatic chippings are seen under the microscope However, in most of the cases (70%), prostatic cancer presents late with advanced disease such as bony metastases. It is an adenocarcinoma arising in the peripheral zone of the gland (which is also the functional part of the gland). The aetiology is unknown. Prostate cancer is now also being identified in asymptomatic men who are found to have a raised PSA (see below) in a routine health check.

On rectal examination the prostate may feel enlarged and "craggy" or a hard nodule may be palpable. The normal mid-line sulcus may be lost. Investigations depend on the patient's age and his symptoms.

If the PSA is raised or clinically the prostate is suspicious, a transrectal ultrasound and biopsy of the prostate should be performed. If a malignancy is diagnosed, the staging procedures include a bone scan and CT scan of the abdomen and pelvis, and a set of liver function tests. If the patient has symptoms of bladder outflow obstruction, then as well as investigating the prostate cancer it is also necessary to perform an ultrasound and urine flow tests, as you would when assessing BPH.

The *stages* of prostatic carcinoma (via the TNM system; outline of the T component of staging):

T0 — no primary tumour identifiable.
T1 — tumour identified incidentally at TURP or with raised PSA.
T2 — palpable tumour without extracapsular extension.
T3 — spread beyond capsule; mobile tumour.
T4 — fixed or locally invasive tumour.

Treatment

TURP can be performed if obstructive symptoms are present, although some of the obstructive symptoms may resolve with hormone treatment. Prostate cancer is driven by androgens, so in patients with metastatic or locally advanced disease the main aim of treatment is to decrease androgen activity. This is achieved by medical or surgical castration. Medical castration can be achieved by LHRH agonists such as Goserelin (Zoladex), which is administered as a monthly subcutaneous injection, or oral antiandrogens such as flutamide or cyproterone. The patients are followed up in the clinic and PSA measurements are used to assess response. There is some evidence that a maximum androgen blockade with an LHRH agonist and an antiandrogen confers some survival advantage. Mean survival once metastases are present is a little over 2½ years.

In early prostate cancer curative treatment by radical prostatectomy or radical radiotherapy is sometimes performed in men under 65 years, but such treatment is highly controversial and the best method of treating early prostate cancer is not known. Radical treatments are offered to patients with localised disease who have a life expectancy of at least 10 years. There is little objective evidence, however, to support the use of any curative treatments.

There is no national screening for prostate cancer. There are several problems regarding prostate cancer screening. The disease is very common, but in many it would not have affected the patient during his life (more than 50% of men over 75 have microfoci at postmortem). An ideal test needs to be found and the best way of treating early prostate cancer needs to be identified. A method of identifying which patients with early prostate cancer will go on to develop metastases is also needed. Until some of these problems are resolved, screening for prostate cancer is inappropriate.

Carcinoma of the Bladder

In Britain almost all (98%) are transitional cell carcinomas (TCC), the remainder being squamous cell carcinomas or adenocarcinomas. In countries with endemic schistosomiasis, squamous cell carcinoma is more common. The aetiology of TCC is unknown, although occupational exposure to chemicals such as aromatic amines and analine dyes has been implicated as carcinogenic. TCC was the first disease for which industrial compensation was awarded. Smoking increases the risk fourfold (nitrosamines are found in cigarette smoke!).

Squamous cell carcinomas are associated with calculi and infections such as schistosomiasis. Adenocarcinomas are associated with persistent urachal remnants.

Carcinoma of the bladder affects males more than females and usually presents with painless haematuria (about 15% present with recurrent UTI's). Urine cytology may identify abnormal cells in the urine, but the diagnosis is usually made by cystoscopy.

Staging is by the TNM system (outline of the T component of staging):

Ta — confined to mucosa.
T1 — tumour invading lamina propria.
T2 — superficial muscle involved.
T3 — deep muscle or perivesical fat involved.
T4 — invasion beyond the bladder into adjacent organs or fixed to the pelvic side wall.

The pathologist also grades them histologically into grades I–III. Grade I means well differentiated and grade III poorly differentiated.

Superficial Bladder Cancers

These can be low grade or high grade Ta or T1 tumours. The low grade superficial tumours are usually exophytic papillary TCC's and about 15% will progress to invasive cancers over 10 years. Treatment is by cystoscopy and diathermy. If no obvious lesion is seen on cystoscopy, multiple biopsies should be taken to exclude carcinoma *in situ* (CIS). High grade (G3) T1 tumours are aggressive and thus need aggressive treatment. Following resection and diathermy there is evidence to suggest benefit from intravesical chemotherapy (e.g. mitomycin) to reduce recurrences. The patients are usually followed up every few months by regular cystoscopies to watch for recurrences. CIS behaves like a high grade TCC and therefore also requires aggressive treatment. Intravesical immunotherapy with BCG can be used to prevent progression of CIS.

Invasive Bladder Cancers

T2 and T3 tumours are treated by either radical radiotherapy or radical cystectomy and formation of an ileal conduit or neobladder out of the small bowel.

T4 disease is treated symptomatically. This may sometimes include cystectomy for intractable bladder symptoms.

RENAL TUMOURS

Renal tumours can be benign or malignant. Cysts are very common in the kidney and are completely benign. Malignant tumours can be primary or secondary, although secondaries in the kidney are unusual. The primary tumours which usually affect those over 50 years old can arise from the kidney substance itself, and are called renal cell carcinomas, or from the lining of the collecting system (in the pelvis or ureters), and are called transitional cell cancers. Other tumours include Wilm's tumour (which affects children) and lymphomas.

Renal cell carcinomas (RCC's) account for more than 80% of renal tumours. These are renal adenocarcinomas (in the past it was thought that they arose from the adrenal rests within the kidney, and hence their old-fashioned name was "hypernephroma"). They actually arise in the renal tubules and are also known as clear cell carcinomas, since the cells appear clear (they are large, with lots of lipids in the cytoplasm). The aetiology is unknown but there is an increased incidence in tobacco smokers. As RCC's grow they become encapsulated by a rim of normal kidney tissue. They can present with haematuria (invasion into the renal pelvis) or with pain (due to presssure effects on local structures and nerves). The classic presentation of an RCC is therefore the triad of pain, haematuria and a renal mass, although this triad is not common and usually the patient has only one or two of these symptoms. RCC's can grow along the renal vein and up the inferior vena cava, and metastases are therefore usually blood-borne and commonly go to the lungs (cannon-ball metastases), bone (pathological fractures), brain, etc. They may present with symptoms due to the production of hormones such as erythropoeitin (polycythaemia) or parathyroid hormone-like substance (hypercalcaemia). Although much loved by the older textbooks, these presentations are in fact quite rare. Nowadays about 50% of RCC's are found incidentally in patients having an ultrasound scan or CT scan for unrelated symptoms.

On examination a mass may be palpable in the loin. *How do you differentiate a kidney from a spleen? The kidney is ballotable (place one hand on the abdomen and the other in the renal angle, raise the hand in the renal angle and keep the other hand still; if you feel a mass touch your upper hand you have balloted a kidney), it moves vertically down on inspiration, and finally it is resonant to percussion (due to the overlying colon). The spleen, on the other hand, has a notch and moves towards the right iliac fossa on inspiration and is dull to percussion.*

If an RCC obstructs the renal vein a varicocoele can result on the left. If you see a varicocoele in the left scrotum, think of an RCC, since the testicular vein on the left drains into the renal vein (it enters the IVC on the right). Only 1% of renal tumours, however, present with a varicocoele.

Diagnosis is usually made on ultrasound, showing a solid mass arising from the kidney. A CT scan is necessary for staging the disease. The other kidney must be checked not only to make sure it is present and functioning, but also because the disease may be bilateral. Treatment is usually by radical nephrectomy (kidney, surrounding fat within Gerota's fascia with or without the adrenal gland). Partial nephrectomy can be considered if the tumour is small or if the patient has a single kidney or poor renal function. Intra-arterial embolisation may be employed to reduce the tumour size preoperatively. Such tumours are resistant to chemotherapy and radiotherapy.

Pelviureteric tumours. These are the same as the transitional cell carcinomas of the bladder, although they account for less than 20% of renal tumours (whereas TCC accounts for almost all of the bladder tumours). They usually present with haematuria. Diagnosis is made by IVU showing a filling defect. Treatment is usually nephrectomy plus removal of the ureter on that side (nephroureterectomy). Follow-up must include regular cystoscopies to look for tumours in the bladder.

A Wilm's tumour (nephroblastoma) contains a bizarre variety of cell and tissue components derived from the mesoderm (for example, as well as kidney substance they may contain fat, cartilage and bone). This is the commonest intra-abdominal tumour in under-10's, with a peak incidence in 2–3-year-olds. It usually presents with a mass, and diagnosis is by ultrasound, CT or MRI. About 10% are bilateral. It is an aggressive, rapidly growing tumour that metastasises often to the lungs. Treatment is usually radical nephrectomy. Chemotherapy is sometimes given postoperatively, depending on the stage. If the tumour is caught early enough, survival is high.

TESTICULAR TUMOURS

Accounting for less than 2% of male malignancies, these are uncommon (despite being the commonest solid tumours in young men). The incidence is about 7 per 100 000 men. Almost all are malignant (95%).

Testicular tumours can be divided into germ cell and non-germ-cell tumours. Almost all are germ cell tumours. The germ cell tumours can be divided into seminomas (40%), teratomas (10%) (also called nonseminomatous germ cell tumours — NSGCT) and mixed (40%). Rarely, choriocarcinomas and yolk sac tumours are seen (these are types of NSGCT).

Non-germ-cell tumours include Leydig cell and Sertoli cell tumours and lymphomas. The Leydig cell and Sertoli cell tumours are very rare; however, they can produce oestrogens and androgens, the symptoms from which usually cause them to present. Lymphomas can occur in the testicle in men in the fifth and sixth decades.

For finals the most important testicular tumours to know about are the seminomas and tertomas. The peak incidence is 20–40 years. 2% are bilateral and there is a significantly increased risk in undescended testes.

Seminomas arise in the epithelium of the seminiferous tubules, tend to grow slowly, and metastasise to regional and para-aortic lymph nodes (remember that the lymphatics usually follow the venous drainage and the testicular veins drain towards the IVC and not to the groin). Placental alkaline phosphatase can be raised in metastatic seminomas.

Teratomas arise from all three germ cell layers, can be more aggressive and carry a poorer prognosis than seminomas. They are subdivided histologically, depending on whether the tumour is well differentiated, moderately differentiated or undifferentiated. The more undifferentiated carry a poorer prognosis. They metastasise via the blood and the lymphatics and most of them secrete βHCG and αFP, which can be used as tumour markers.

Staging of Testicular Tumours

(I)   Tumour confined to testis.
(II)   Involvement of lymph nodes below diaphragm.
(III) Lymph nodes above diaphragm involved.
(IV)   Extralymphatic spread.

The tumours usually present as a painless testicular mass, although they can present with a secondary hydrocoele or a painful lump. They may be misdiagnosed initially as a epididymo-orchitis. On examination you should look for evidence of lymphatic spread (abdominal, supraclaviular and chest).

A common exam question concerns how to examine a scrotum. You should always ask yourself four questions: Is the lump in the testis or is it separate, can I get above it (you should be able to get above a testicular lesion, but not a hernia), is the testis tender, and does it transilluminate? A hard mass in the testis, which you can get above and which does not transilluminate, should raise your suspicions.

An ultrasound can be performed to see if a scrotal lump is connected with the testis and if it is solid or cystic. A solid lump suggests malignancy. Serum αFP (never raised in seminomas) and βHCG should be sent, as should placental alkaline phosphatase. To stage the disease a CT scan of the chest, abdomen and pelvis is performed.

Treatment starts by an orchidectomy via a groin incision. The reason for the groin incision is threefold: to allow the cord to be clamped before mobilising the testicle, to prevent seeding the scrotal skin, and to allow the incision to be within the radiotherapy field. The testis is then brought out and examined. If the lump appears malignant (or a frozen section is done), then it is excised together with the spermatic cord. Further treatment depends on the tumour type, and its stage and grade. Tumour markers should again be sent off at one week, since if they are still high after surgery this indicates that metastases are present.

Seminomas are very radiosensitive. Radiotherapy is usually given both to the groin and to the abdominal lymph nodes. Stage IV tumours are usually given chemotherapy initially, although they are rare (as seminomas usually present earlier than teratomas). Teratomas are less sensitive to radiotherapy, and combination chemotherapy (for example actinomycin, bleomycin, methotrexate and cisplatin) is usually given at the start.

The prognosis for Stage I seminomas and teratomas is extremely good (96–100% five-year survival) and for Stage IV disease five-year survival is 55–75%, depending on the tumour and the tumour bulk. Any recurrence following initial treatment is likely to occur within the first 18–24 months and close surveillance is therefore very important over this period, with repeat CT scanning and tumour markers, initially every six weeks and then every three months.

OTHER CONDITIONS OF THE TESTES

Hydrocoele. This is fluid around the testis in the tunica vaginalis. The condition can be primary or secondary. Primary (idiopathic) hydrocoeles (the vast majority) develop slowly and can become large and tense. They are commonest in the over-40 age group, although they can occur

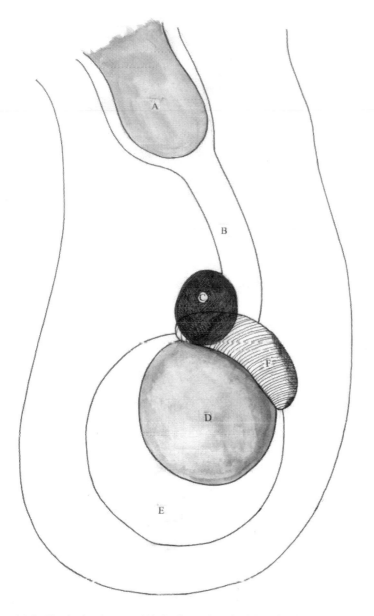

Figure 14.1. Testicular lumps. (A) Indirect inguinal hernia, (B) spermatic cord, (c) epididymal cyst, (D) testis, (E) Hydrocoele, (F) epididymis.

in children. If you recall your embryology the testis descends from the abdomen taking a layer of peritoneum with it called the processus vaginalis. Normally the sac is sealed off; however, if it remains patent fluid can form in it, causing a primary hydrocoele (if bowel contents enter the sac, then this is an infantile hernia; treatment of the infant hydrocoele is the same as that for an infantile hernia). Primary hydrocoeles can develop in adults in the absence of a patent processus. Secondary hydrocoeles are usually secondary to trauma, infection or malignancy. In contrast they develop rapidly, are not tense and may contain blood.

On examination the testis is usually impalpable, you can get above the swelling (which has a smooth surface), and it transilluminates brilliantly. An ultrasound should be performed to look at the testis. A small hydrocoele may not need treatment if the patient is not bothered by it. Larger hydrocoeles can be tapped but the fluid (which is straw-coloured) will invariably return. Definitive surgical treatment involves either plicating the tunica vaginalis (Lord's repair) or inverting the sac (Jaboulay's repair).

Epididymo-orchitis. This is inflammation of the testis and epididymis due to infection. The young are more susceptible to viral infections (e.g. mumps), the old to bacterial infections (e.g. *E. coli* following a UTI), and the sexually active to chlamydial and gonococcal infection. The typical presentation is acute onset of severe testicular pain. The patient may feel unwell with fever, have a urethral discharge and symptoms of a UTI. Pain may be referred to the right iliac fossa. On examination the testis is tender, red and warm. You can often feel a markedly swollen epididymis separate from the testicle. If you place your hand under the scrotum and elevate it, this sometimes relieves the pain of epididymo-orchitis, but not of torsion.

Testicular torsion. This can affect any age but is most common between the ages of 12 and 27; it can occur, rarely, in neonates. There is a higher incidence in undescended testes. It is a urological emergency, as the testis will infarct within hours if the torsion is not treated. The testis twists within the tunica vaginalis and the blood supply is compromised. It usually presents in the same way as epididymo-orchitis (usually without the UTI symptoms). On examination the testis may lie horizontally and be retracted compared to the other side.

The main difficulty when seeing a patient with a tender painful scrotum is in differentiating between epididymo-orchitis and torsion. Patients with epididymo-orchitis may have a longer history and may have urethritis with burning pain on micturition. An MSU should be dipstixed and sent urgently for microscopy, as this may help in cases where infection is likely. However, if you are in any doubt, then surgical exploration is essential. If you explore it and it is an infection no harm is done, but if you treat a torsion conservatively the testicle will die. When you are exploring a testicle for torsion, the patient must always be warned of the possibility of orchidectomy if the testicle has infarcted. At the time of surgery both testicles are fixed to ensure they cannot twist in the future. Doppler ultrasound is quite good at showing the integrity of the arterial blood flow to the testis, but should not delay surgical exploration.

RENAL COLIC

Stones may form at any level of the urinary tract. Symptoms depend on the site of stone impaction. The pain is due to the peristalsis proximal to the obstruction. The size of the stone is not correlated with the amount of pain, as a large staghorn calculus of the renal pelvis may be painless and a tiny stone in the ureter may be agonizing. The classic story is sudden onset of severe pain that makes the patient writhe about in agony, unable to get comfortable (in contrast with the pain of peritonism, where the patient lies still). The patient is sweaty, nauseous and may vomit. A stone in the ureter usually causes pain which starts in the loin and radiates down into the groin. There may also be pain in the scrotum or labia. A stone in the bladder may cause stranguary (desire to pass something that will not pass). A stone in the mid ureter may mimic appendicitis on the right and diverticulitis on the left.

Most cases are calcium stones (80%) complexed with oxalate (35%), phosphate (3%) or mixed oxalate and phosphate crystals (40%). Others include struvite (magnesium aluminium phosphate), cysteine, urate and xanthine. They usually form when there is a high concentration of solutes in the urine, especially in dehydration. Although in some there is a familial tendency, the exact reason why stones form is often unclear. The calcium stones may rarely be associated with hyperparathyroidism, renal tubular acidosis and medullary sponge kidney. The phosphate containing stones (especially the struvite) are associated with urinary tract infections, especially *proteus*, which breaks down urea to form ammonia and alkaline urine, which precipitates these stones. In contrast, acid urine tends to precipitate the calcium oxalate and urate containing stones.

90% of renal stones are radio-opaque (urate stones are translucent), in contrast to gallstones, where 90% are radio-lucent.

Examination is usually normal, although the patient may have tenderness in the renal angle especially on percussion, which indicates retroperitoneal inflammation. A urine dipstix should reveal haematuria (in 90% of cases) and this should be confirmed by microscopy. If the urine shows no blood you should be thinking of alternative diagnoses. These include an abdominal aortic aneurysm, appendicitis, pyelonephritis, diverticulitis and gynaecological causes.

Analgesia should be given once the diagnosis is suspected. The pain from ureteric colic is usually alleviated by nonsteroidal anti-inflammatory agents. An IVU is performed, usually by the casualty doctor. A baseline KUB X-ray is taken first. You should know the normal course of the ureters. They start at the renal pelvis, which lies at the level of L1 (look for the 12th rib, which is joined to T12, and go down one vertebra). They travel down from here along the line of the transverse processes towards the sacroiliac joint (where they cross over the iliac vessels). At this point they travel backwards towards the ischial spines and then forwards into the bladder. The common sites for obstruction to occur are the pelviureteric junction, the SIJ, where the ureter crosses over the iliac vessels, and the vesicoureteric junction (VUJ). Remember that phleboliths (calcification in veins) are common in this region, but they are usually multiple, more rounded and have a radioluscent centre.

A venflon is inserted and the radiopaque contrast is injected into the arm. A film is taken after 5 min and another postmicturition. If there is any abnormality on the IVU, then a delayed film after about an hour is usually taken. Further films should be taken until contrast is seen down to the level of obstruction. Request films at 1, 2, 4, 8 and 24 h if necessary. In the normal kidney, contrast is seen flowing towards the bladder. The ureter is a hollow tube that peristalses six times a minute. Students often get confused, because they see some contrast in the ureter and then see what looks like a stricture and think this must be a block. Actually this simply represents a wave of peristalsis and is normal. If there is a block what you see is a standing column of contrast above the stone. The renal pelvis may be dilated and there may be blunting of the calyces. If there is complete obstruction on one side you may see a dense nephrogram (the kidney outline is visibly radiopaque), with no contrast entering the ureter.

If the patient is known to be pregnant, asthmatic or atopic, then an IVU might be contraindicated and an ultrasound may be performed (or he can be admitted for an IVU under steroid cover).

If the pain resolves and the kidney is not obstructed on IVU, the patient should be allowed to go home with oral analgesia and an appointment for the urology clinic. If the pain persists or the kidney is obstructed, he should be admitted. If he has an obstructed kidney and develops a fever, particularly with loin pain, then this is a urological emergency, as damage to the kidney can occur if it is not drained urgently. Antibiotics should be started and urgent arrangements made to insert a nephrostomy tube to drain the kidney percutaneously.

Routine bloods should be sent to assess renal function; screening for calcium, urate and phosphate levels may be helpful in the case of recurrent episodes. The urine may be sieved to catch the stone as it passes and a 24 h urine collection may be analysed, as this may give information on ways to avoid a recurrence in the future.

90% of stones less than 4 mm in size pass spontaneously and about half of stones up to 7 mm pass spontaneously. Conservative management is therefore first line in such patients. The urine is sieved and the patients are given analgesia and encouraged to drink a lot. Stones greater than 7 mm do not tend to pass and intervention is likely to be needed.

The treatment of renal and ureteric stones depends on the size and position of the stone. Extracorporeal shock wave lithotripsy (ESWL) is the treatment of choice for most renal and ureteric stones. In the middle third of the ureter it is often difficult to visualise the stone, due to the overlying iliac bone or sacrum; however, ESWL can still sometimes be used by adjusting the position of the patient. ESWL can be performed on a day case or out-patient basis. Lithotripters use piezoelectrically generated shock waves to shatter the stone, under image-intensifying control. Other techniques for removing a stone include ureteroscopy, where the stone is visualised by passing a fine endoscope up the ureter and then captured in a wire basket or fragmented with a pneumatic instrument (called a lithoclast) or with a laser.

If the stone is in the renal pelvis and is too large for lithotripsy, then percutaenous removal may be necessary. Under ultrasound or fluoroscopic guidance a needle is inserted into the calyx of the kidney. A guide wire is passed down the needle and into the ureter, and the needle is then removed. A series of dilators are inserted over the guide wire to create a track to the renal pelvis. The stone is then fragmented under direct vision and the fragments are removed (percutaneous nephrolithotomy).

In summary, ESWL is used for stones less than 2 cm in size in the kidney. If the stone is larger than 2 cm or if there is calyceal obstruction, then percutaneous removal may be necessary. For stones in the upper third of the ureter, ESWL is used. For stones in the lower third of the ureter, ureteroscopy can be used. The middle third of the ureter is a difficult region, as it may be a difficult target for ESWL and too high for retrograde ureteroscopy, although the stone can sometimes be pushed back up the ureter and then treated with ESWL. In difficult cases, for example an impacted ureteric stone, open surgery is occasionally indicated.

PAEDIATRIC UROLOGY

At birth adhesions are present between the glans and the foreskin and the prepuce normally becomes retractile by the age of two. Sometimes the parents notice the prepuce "ballooning" up when the child micturates, due to urine collecting in the space between foreskin and glans, before escaping through the narrow opening. This is normal and the parents should be advised not to force the foreskin back, otherwise a *phimosis* can result, which is a narrowing of the opening of the foreskin. A phimosis can also result secondary to infection and, in an adult, may cause painful intercourse. It is usually treated by circumcision. (A *paraphimosis* is a swelling of the glans and is caused by a tight foreskin being retracted and not replaced. This can occur after catheterisation. The tight foreskin blocks the venous return and the glans becomes oedematous and swollen. This is usually treated by reducing the oedema with compression, squeezing the foreskin and glans with a cupped hand. The glans is then pressed in whilst trying to flip the foreskin forwards to its normal position.)

Hypospadias. This is an abnormal position of the urethral opening, due to failure of development. The urethra can open anywhere on the ventral (undersurface) surface of the penis. Repair is usually carried out by paediatric surgeons.

Undescended testes. In 80% of cases the undescended testis is palpable in the inguinal canal. If the testis is palpable in the inguinal canal or at the top of the scrotum, orchidopexy is performed (the testis is fixed in the scrotum, usually by mobilising the testis and placing it between the dartos muscle and the skin). This should be done by the age of 18 months, to prevent damage to the testis (spontaneous descent is rare after one year). After the age of two, the testis is likely to be damaged and incapable of spermatogenesis.

Complete absence of the testis is uncommon (check notes to see if present at birth check), and if it is not palpable it should be assumed to be intra-abdominal and CT or MRI may be needed to locate it.

If an undescended testicle presents after puberty, many urologists would advocate location and removal of the testicle because of the risk of malignant change.

15

ORTHOPAEDICS

Orthopaedics is a large subject that cannot be covered in its entirety within the scope of this book. We have therefore attempted to deal with general fracture management and topics that are commonly asked about. You should know how to examine the hand, hip, knee and shoulder with fluency and should practise these examinations on patients and on friends before the exam, so that they become second nature.

EXAMINATION OF THE HIP

Orthopaedic surgeons tend to use four-letter words, and the orthopaedic examination is therefore easily remembered as: LOOK, FEEL, MOVE and X-RAY. Always examine the abnormal or painful areas last. In a viva, always ask the patient whether he minds your examining him, and whether he has any pain (in a similar way to checking your mirrors in a driving test, make sure the examiners note that you have done so). Likewise, observe his face for pain, because hurting your patient is one of the biggest errors you can make in the exam.

Pain arising from the hip joint is often felt in the groin or anterior thigh, and sometimes it is referred down to the knee. If the pain is predominantly in the back of the hip, it is usually referred from the lumbar spine. It is true to say that pains are usually referred distally, and so a knee pain may be coming from the hip and a hip pain may be coming from the back, etc.

The method of examination will differ, depending on the circumstances. For example, an elderly lady seen in casualty after a fall will be assessed on a trolley with her supine, and a young patient may walk into your surgery and assessment of gait will therefore be noted initially. Make sure that the hips and the entire legs are exposed.

On *inspection* look at the *attitude* or *posture* of the patient and the limbs; for example, the leg may be shortened and externally rotated in a hip fracture. Look for any obvious scars (do not forget to check the back of the hip), swelling or wasting of the quadriceps, glutei or hamstrings. Inspect the legs for signs of venous or arterial disease (this will be important if an operation is being considered) and examine for any leg length discrepancy. You should differentiate between real shortening (loss of bone length) and apparent shortening (due to a deformity of the pelvic or hip position). First try to position the pelvis so that the anterior superior iliac spines (ASIS) are at the same level. You will now observe any obvious differences by comparing the level of the knees and of the ankles.

On *palpation* measure the distance from the ASIS to the medial malleolus on each side (true length) and the distance from a fixed point such as the xiphisternum (or umbilicus) to the medial malleolus (apparent length). The apparent length will be shorter if the pelvis is tilted upwards. Feel the bony contours, including the greater trochanter, the ASIS, the iliac crests and the pubic rami.

Test *movement* passively and actively. Normal ranges for the hip are: flexion (0–130), extension (usually in a prone position, 0–10), abduction (0–45), adduction (0–30), external rotation (0 45) and internal rotation (0–20). To test rotation, flex the knee to 90°, and put one hand on the knee and the other on the foot — remember that external rotation brings the foot medially. To test adduction the limb is crossed over the opposite limb. Power should be recorded for each muscle group. One problem with the hip is that limitation of movement can be obscured by movement of the pelvis and hence a gross limitation of extension can be masked by arching the back into excessive lordosis. Therefore, when describing the range of motion always comment on any fixed flexion deformities first. You can use *Thomas's test* to check for this — fully flex the two hips simultaneously to obliterate the lumbar lordosis (you can place one hand under the lower back to confirm this). Whilst holding one leg in this position, ask the patient to straighten the other leg as fully as possible. The angle between the thigh and the bed is the fixed flexion deformity (the cause is often osteoarthritis). Repeat the test on the other side.

The function and stability of the hip can be assessed by *Trendelenburg's test*. Ask the patient to stand on one leg by bending at the knee (not at the hip — as if he were doing an impression of a pirate with a wooden leg!). The normal pelvis tilts upwards on the unsupported side by contraction of the abductors on the weight-bearing side. A positive Trendelenburg sign occurs when the pelvis droops on the unsupported side — "*sound side sags*". The causes of a positive test are weakness of the abductors, dislocation or fracture of the hip and any painful condition of the hip.

Gait involves all the joints of the lower limb, and it is therefore difficult sometimes to discern the cause of an abnormal gait. If the patient limps because of pain, then this is called *antalgic gait*. Here the weight-bearing (stance) phase on the affected side is shorter, as the patient tries to avoid putting weight onto the affected side. The commonest cause is osteoarthritis.

In finals, at the end of the exam you are usually asked if there is anything else you would like to do, and it is probably acceptable to say "I would also like to examine the leg pulses and neurological system" at that point rather than do it routinely, as time is short and you want to give an impression of succinctness.

Incidentally, if you see a case in finals where the leg is deformed with asymmetrical muscular wasting and sensation is entirely normal, always look around the room for a caliper or cast brace, as polio cases often feature in finals (despite the fact that we see almost no new cases in this country!).

EXAMINATION OF THE KNEE

There are three components to the knee joint: the medial and lateral compartments (between the femoral condyles and the tibial plateau) and the patellofemoral compartment. The joint surfaces are lined by articular cartilage (which becomes worn in osteoarthritis). In addition there are the two C-shaped cartilaginous menisci lining the medial and lateral compartments. There are two parallel ligaments running in opposite directions at the centre of the knee, which help make it stable, and they are called the cruciate ligaments. The anterior cruciate stops the tibia moving anteriorly on the femur, whereas the posterior cruciate stops the tibia moving backwards on the femur. The capsule encloses the knee joint and is strengthened on the medial and lateral sides by the medial and lateral collateral ligaments.

As mentioned above, gait can be tested at the beginning or at the end of the examination — it does not really matter, as long as you remember it. With the patient standing, look at the alignment checking for valgus (*knock knees* — deviation of the distal part away from the mid-line) or varus deformities at the knees. *Look* at the foot arches for flat feet (pes planus), which can contribute to knee pathology. Look at the position of the patellae — are they symmetrical? Look for quadriceps wasting (which implies lack of use), any visible scars or obvious effusions to the knees (even a small effusion may be noted by the absence of the normal hollow on either side of the patella).

Feel the skin temperature. This is helpful in the knee as the joint is superficial (unlike the hip); always comparing with the opposite side. To test for an effusion you can use the patella tap or stroke test. To perform the *patella tap*, compress the suprapatellar pouch with your left hand and press down gently on the patella with the fingers of your right hand. You should be able to bounce the patella up and down on the fluid, always comparing that to the other side. If there is only a small effusion a better test is the *stroke test*, where you empty the medial compartment by massaging the fluid into the lateral side of the knee. Then apply gentle pressure over the lateral side, just above the patella, and watch the gutter on the medial side. It will balloon up with the fluid you have pushed over if there is an effusion.

Palpate the bones, testing for localized tenderness (patella, tibial tuberosity and joint edges of the distal femur and tibia). Feel along the medial and lateral collateral ligaments for tenderness, and with the knee flexed to 90° you can feel the joint space (tenderness here implies synovial or meniscal pathology). The popliteal fossa should be examined for a popliteal cyst and a pulsatile popliteal aneurysm. A popliteal cyst is a nontender fluctuant lump that follows either synovial rupture or herniation. If there is underlying joint pathology such as osteoarthritis, then it is called a Baker's cyst.

Do not confuse a popliteal cyst or aneurysm (which are in the midline) with an enlarged semimembranosus bursa, which is on the medial side between semimembranosus and the medial head of gastrocnemius and is often more prominent in a straight knee.

Movement should be tested actively and passively, and for the knee it is essentially flexion and extension, comparing the two sides. Note any fixed flexion deformities at the knee — if you can passively fully straighten the knee then it is not a fixed deformity! During the passive movements of the knee you should place one hand over the front of the knee, feeling for crepitus (implying irregular patellofemoral movement, usually due to wearing of the articular cartilage, i.e. chondromalacia). You can test side-to-side movements of the patella (if the patella has dislocated in the past, the patient often becomes anxious and is not keen on this — this is called patella apprehension).

To test the *collateral ligaments* flex the knee slightly (about 30°) and apply valgus and varus stress to the knee joint to see if there is any laxity, which implies a tear (you cannot test this in full extension as the knee "locks").

To test the *menisci* you can perform *McMurray's test*. Flex the knee as far as possible. Then grasp the joint line between the thumb and fingers of one hand and use the other hand to internally and externally rotate the foot (to load pressure onto the medial and lateral menisci respectively) as the knee is slowly extended. If there is a torn piece of cartilage between the articular surfaces in the knee, you may feel or hear a click as it is set free. Always look at the patient's face for pain and grimacing.

To test the *cruciates*, have the patient lie flat, and flex the knee to 90°. Look from the side for any sag of the tibia in relation to the femur. This implies a tear of the posterior cruciate. Now anchor the foot by sitting on it and grab the leg just below the knee with both hands and push backwards (*posterior draw test* — for a posterior cruciate tear) and then pull forwards (*anterior draw test* — for a tear of the anterior cruciate). If the tibia moves forwards more on one side when compared to the other leg, then this is likely to be a positive draw test, implying a rupture of the anterior cruciate ligament (beware if there was a posterior sag, since you may simply be correcting this rather than testing the anterior cruciate). A modification of this test is the *Lachman test*, where the knee is flexed only to 30°, the left hand grasps the thigh and the right hand grasps the tibia just below the knee. As the thigh is held still the tibia is pulled anteriorly, again testing the anterior cruciate. You do need big hands for this test, although it is said to be a much more sensitive test than the anterior draw. One final test for the anterior cruciate rupture is the *pivot shift test*, which reproduces the instability that the patient experiences when his leg gives way. Flex the knee fully and hold the internally rotated foot with one hand (right hand if testing the right side). Apply a slight valgus strain to the knee with the opposite hand as you slowly extend it fully. In a positive test you will feel a click as the tibia shifts anteriorly falling into place, when the knee is extended. In the authors' experience these tests are all best learnt by direct demonstration rather than from a textbook.

EXAMINATION OF THE SHOULDER

Pain in the region of the shoulder may be referred from the cervical spine, the chest and mediastinum, and from irritation of the diaphragm. The shoulder is the most mobile of all joints and it therefore has to sacrifice some stability. The rotator cuff has four muscles (supraspinatus, infraspinatus, teres minor and subscapularis) that surround the joint holding the humeral head in against the glenoid providing some stability, although they are deficient inferiorly which is therefore a site of potential weakness.

Expose the whole torso, and observe for bruises, redness and scars. Look from the front and then ask the patient to turn around, and inspect from behind, comparing the two sides, looking for asymmetry, position of the arms, wasting of the deltoid or pectoral muscles and prominence of the acromioclavicular joint (ACJ). Do not forget to inspect the axilla.

Feel the temperature and for any localized tenderness (sternoclavicular joint, the clavicle, spine of scapula, acromion process, ACJ, humeral head and greater and lesser tuberosities).

Movement is again active and passive. Ask the patient to abduct both arms until the fingers point upwards. Watch his face for grimacing and note which part of the arc is painful. Pain in mid-range of movement is usually due to rotator cuff pathology, such as inflammation or a tear of the supraspinatus. Pain at the end of abduction may be due to acromioclavicular osteoarthritis.

If you recall your anatomy, you can only abduct to about 90°, after which the greater tuberosity hits the glenoid and you need to externally rotate the arm to complete the abduction. The scapula also rotates. Observe movement at the glenohumeral joint and of the scapula on both sides. Test also flexion, extension, rotation and adduction (the arm moves in front of the body). Active rotation is best tested by asking the patient to touch the back of his neck with both hands (external rotation in abduction) and the small of his back (internal rotation). Now passively repeat all of these movements. Passive rotation is tested with the elbow touching the side of the body and flexed to 90°. Bringing the hand across the body is internal rotation; away from the body, external rotation. Record the power of each muscle group and test for any neurovascular deficit in both arms.

Test for winging of the scapulae by asking the patient to place his hands out in front of him and press against a wall. If the serratus anterior (which normally holds the scapula against the chest wall) is paralysed, then the scapula will protrude like a wing. This is usually due to damage to the nerve to the serratus anterior (long thoracic nerve of Bell).

There are many special tests that can be performed on the shoulder; however, you probably just need to know the above for finals purposes.

A terribly rare inherited disorder is craniocleidodysostosis, where there is absence of the clavicles and the patient can bring both shoulders to the mid-line. This is the sort of rare but interesting case that sometimes turns up at finals, so it is probably worth a mention.

EXAMINATION OF THE HANDS

This a very common short case in finals (usually with respect to rheumatoid hands), appearing in the medicine section of the exam. Although you may still see a rheumatoid hand in surgical finals you are more likely to see a nerve injury, Dupuytren's, trigger finger or a ganglion. As hand examination is covered well in the rheumatology books, you will simply find a summary of the examination here. Before we start, it my help you to think for second or two about the following fact: the thumb, the index finger and the middle finger are the most important for the functioning of the hand (touch, grip, precise movements), whereas the ring finger and the little finger are more important for grip strength.

Introduce yourself and ask the patient whether he minds your examining his hands and whether they are painful. If a pillow is available place it under the hands for comfort.

Note the following (distal interphalangeal joints = DIPJ's; proximal interphalangeal joints = PIPJ's; metacarpophalangeal joints = MCPJ's):

- You should refer to the fingers as index, middle, ring and little and not 1, 2, 3, etc.
- The DIPJ's are flexed by the flexor digitorum profundus (inserting into the base of the distal phalanx) and the PIPJ's are flexed by the flexor digitorum superficialis (inserting into the base of the middle phalanx).
- The flexor digitorum profundus (FDP) is innervated by both the median and ulna nerves, usually the median nerve supplying the part that flexes the index and middle fingers, with the ulna nerve supplying the part that flexes the ring and little fingers.
- The Palmar interrossei ADduct the fingers (PAD), whereas the Dorsal interrossei ABduct or spread the fingers (DAB). The interrossei and lumbricals are responsible for the movement of flexion at the MCPJ's (whilst the PIPJ's and DIPJ's are extended).
- All of the intrinsic muscles of the hand are supplied by T1 as the ulnar nerve [except the LOAF muscles (see under "carpal tunnel syndrome"), which are supplied by the median nerve].

Inspect the hands, look at the dorsum and then ask the patient to turn his hands over so that you can look at the palms. Look for any scars, palmar erythema, muscle wasting, nail changes or obvious deformities [Dupuytren's contracture; mallet finger; Boutonniere, swan neck, Z thumb deformities and Heberden's nodes (which are nodular swellings at the DIPJ's, seen in osteoarthritis); note that primary osteoarthritis tends to affect the DIPJ's whereas RA tends to affect the MCPJ's and PIPJ's, sparing the DIPJ's].

Feel the temperature, and palpate all of the individual joints (especially the MCPJ's), feeling for any synovial or capsular thickening or swelling (indicative of active synovitis).

Ask the patient to make a fist and then to touch the thumb to the tip of each finger (opposition). Then test finger abduction and adduction. Test the strength of each of these muscle groups by asking him to grasp your finger in a grip and to stop you pulling your fingers out from between his opposed thumb and little finger. Test resisted abduction by asking him to keep his fingers spread against resistance, and resisted adduction by asking him to grip a piece of paper between his adducted fingers as you pull it out.

Test sensation in the median (the tip of the index finger), radial (the dorsum of the base of the thumb) and ulna (the tip of the little finger) nerve distributions. As to testing the nerve function in more detail, see the section on nerve injuries at the end of the chapter.

Finally, test function by asking the patient to do up a shirt button, hold an object such as a key or a pen, etc.

If when the fingers are extended (from a grip) one of the fingers stays flexed but can be straightened by the patient (usually with a snap), this is likely to be a trigger finger (usually caused by thickening of the fibrous tendon sheath, perhaps due to repetitive trauma).

FRACTURE CLASSIFICATION AND MANAGEMENT

A fracture is a break in the continuity of a bone. It should be thought of as a soft tissue injury around a broken bone, since more problems arise from the soft tissue damage than from the fracture itself.

Fractures can be open or closed, intra or extra-articular, and displaced or undisplaced. Open fractures (also called "compound") are fractures where the surface wound communicates with the fracture and there is thus potential for contamination through the wound (the wound does not necessarily have to be skin and may be an internal body surface, such as a lung). Closed fractures (they used to be called "simple", but this is not a very good name since many are far from simple) are fractures where the skin remains intact. You cannot tell from an X-ray whether a fracture is open or closed.

Types of Fracture

Types of fracture include transverse, oblique, spiral, comminuted (multifragmentary, i.e. more than two fragments), *avulsion* (caused by a traction force, a bony fragment being torn off by a tendon or ligament), *compression* (or *crush*, which occurs when cancellous bone is crumpled, such as in the calcaneum after a fall from a height or in the vertebral bodies, especially in the elderly) and *stress fractures* (these occur after repeated stresses that cause fatigue to bone, often seen in athletes, usually in the lower limbs). Two other types you need to know about are greenstick and pathological fractures.

Greenstick fractures are seen in children, whose bones are softer and more pliable and tend to bend rather than break. The cortex on one side tends to buckle (imagine bending a branch of a green twig).

Pathological fractures are fractures occurring in a bone that has already been weakened by disease, and may occur at normal physiological stresses. There are many causes, including generalized bone diseases or metastatic deposits in the bone. One could think of pathological fractures as being of two types: one where a fracture occurs in a patient with generalized bone disease, such as a crushed vertebra or a fractured neck of femur in an osteoporotic lady; the other type occurs in patients with normal bone structure, but the fracture is in a localised area of abnormal bone, such as through a metastatic deposit.

Osteoporosis is the commonest cause of pathological fracture, especially in the spine and femoral neck. Although most books tend to

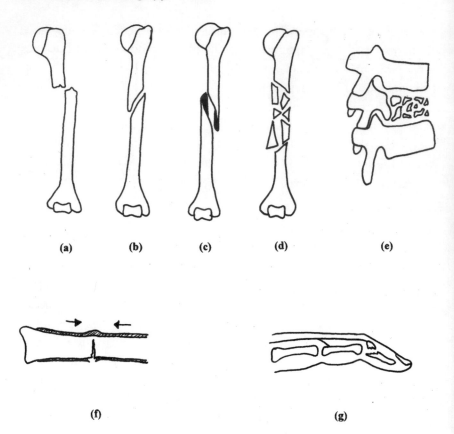

Figure 15.1. Types of fracture. (a) Transverse, (b) oblique, (c) spiral, (d) comminuted, (e) crush, (f) greenstick, (g) avulsion.

classify osteoporotic fractures as pathological, in practice we do not tend to refer to them as being pathological, otherwise most of the fractures in the geriatric age group would be "pathological", and this term is therefore usually reserved for those involving malignancies.

Displacement of Fractures

When the bone breaks, the fragments often are displaced due to the force of the injury and also due to gravity and the pull of the muscles

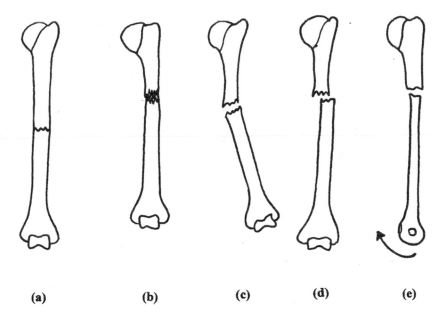

(a)   (b)   (c)   (d)   (e)

Figure 15.2. Displacement of fractures. (a) Undisplaced, (b) impacted, (c) angulated (25°), (d) lateral displacement (50%), (e) rotation.

attached to the fragments. There are many terms used to describe displacement, such as "impaction", "angulation", "opposition" and "rotation". Impaction implies that the fragments are driven into one another, causing shortening. Angulation (or alignment) means that one fragment is angulated in relation to the other, which if left alone may lead to deformity of the limb. Angulation is described in degrees.

Dislocations. This is a *complete loss* of congruity between the articulating surfaces of a joint. The term implies disruption to the capsule and soft tissues around the joint. Dislocations should be relocated as soon as possible, to prevent long term complications.

Subluxation. This is *partial loss* of contact between two joint surfaces, as is seen for example at the acromioclavicular joint. Both dislocations and subluxations can be associated with fractures, and they are then termed "fracture dislocations" or "fracture subluxations".

Fracture Healing

There are five stages to the healing of a fracture. We *bleed* into the fracture and an inflammatory reaction is set up, the cells *proliferate*, and early bone and cartilage is formed (*callus*), which then *consolidates* (as woven bone is transformed into stronger lamellar bone). The bone then *remodels* to the normal stresses it is placed under, and over a period of months to years the bone returns to its normal shape.

The rate of repair depends on many factors, including which bone is affected, the position and blood supply of the fragments, the age and general health of the patient, and the method of restriction of the fracture (plaster Vs surgery).

As a rough guide, however, the long bones of a healthy adult's upper limb take about 6 weeks to heal and the lower limb about 12 weeks. Hence, upper limb fractures usually have a plaster on for about 6 weeks. Children heal quicker and for them you can probably halve these times.

DESCRIBING A FRACTURE ON AN X-RAY

X-rays must always have two views taken at 90° to each other (usually an AP and a lateral X-ray), and as a rule they should include both the joint above and the joint below the fracture. If an X-ray is taken of a long bone, such as the femur, the entire bone should be on one X-ray. Thus if you are given one view of an X-ray in the exam, before you make any comment on the X-ray your first statement should be "May I see another view?", followed by "May I see an X-ray of the joint above and below the fracture?"

When you are given an X-ray and asked to describe a fracture, you should describe the affected part of the body (e.g. the limb), the affected bone or bones, the type of fracture (open, closed, intra-articular or extra-articular) and its displacement.

An example: *These are AP and lateral X-rays of the right forearm of Mrs Jane Smith, taken on the 5th of March. They show an oblique extra-articular fracture of the distal radius, which is impacted and therefore shortened, and there is about 10° of radial and dorsal angulation of the distal fragment. There is also an associated undisplaced fracture of the ulnar styloid. This injury is known as Colles' fracture.*

If asked about management of a fracture, even if you do not know much about this type of fracture, simply describe it on the X-ray and discuss management in terms of the four R's (see below).

MANAGEMENT OF FRACTURES

These are the four R's:
(1) Resuscitation
(2) Reduction
(3) Restriction (immobilization)
(4) Rehabilitation

(1) Resuscitation

Following the ATLS® guidelines (see Chapter 4), one should deal with associated life-threatening injuries first. The airway, breathing and circulation take priority over the fracture. In the case of any major trauma, the standard trauma series of X-rays should be performed as part of the ATLS® primary survey. These include a C-spine, a chest and a pelvic X-ray.

The fracture is usually assessed in the secondary survey, unless it is a bleeding open wound, in which case a sterile pressure dressing is applied during the primary survey, under C for circulation, as would be an unstable pelvic fracture.

Once this is done and you are assessing the fracture, you should note the condition of the skin and soft tissues, check for any neurovascular deficit and examine the associated joints before any X-rays are taken.

Open fractures are managed differently from closed fractures. The life-threatening injuries are dealt with first in the same way but, because of the risk of infection, they are booked for theatre as an emergency (within six hours). The wound should be swabbed and any gross contaminants should be removed. Antibiotics should be started (for example, a broad spectrum cephalosporin) and a tetanus booster given if needed (a toxoid booster lasts ten years). A photograph should be taken so that the wound does not need to be inspected repeatedly, and then the wound should be covered with an iodine-soaked dressing. The limb is usually immobilized using a splint to prevent pain and further contamination whilst awaiting theatre. If there is gross deformity, manipulation under sedation may be needed before it can be splinted. The neurovascular status must be checked both before and after this is carried out.

The patient is booked for examination under anaesthesia (EUA). When he is anaesthetized the wound is thoroughly washed out and any contaminated or dead tissue is debrided. The fracture is assessed and stabilized either by internal fixation or an external fixator.

If the wound is large and primary closure is unlikely to be achieved, then a plastic surgeon should ideally be present in theatre, as it may be possible to perform a skin graft or flap procedure (alternatively the wound can be left open and reinspected at about 48 h for delayed primary closure or a plastics procedure). Remember the saying "In open fractures — save life, save limb and stabilize fracture".

Other fractures that need urgent treatment include fracture dislocations and those fractures with vascular or neurological compromise.

(2) Reduction

Not all fractures require reduction, either because there is no displacement or because the displacement that is there will not affect the final result. An example of a fracture that is not usually reduced is a fracture of the clavicle, as normal function will be restored without intervention. It is really a balance between function and acceptable appearance.

If a fracture is displaced and left in that position, the bones may not unite, but if they do unite the position may be unacceptable, with resultant deformity. Alignment of the fracture is more important than opposition.

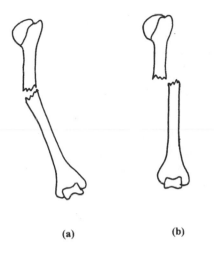

(a)   (b)

Figure 15.3. Alignment of a fracture. (a) Well opposed but angulated; (b) well aligned but poorly opposed (more acceptable than (a)).

Methods of Reduction

(I)   *Manipulation* (or closed reduction). This is usually under local, regional or general anaesthetic. The distal fragment is pulled in the line of the bone to disimpact the fragments, and the bones are then repositioned manually.

(II) *Traction.* This is used when the contraction forces of large muscles need to be overcome, particularly for fractures of the femur. Traction can be effected by using the skin (skin traction) or by using the bones (skeletal traction). With skin traction, adhesive tape applied to the skin holds the frame. With skeletal traction a pin is placed through a bone distal to the fracture. In either case the limb is pulled, usually via a pulley system, in the direction of a weight applied at the end of the bed.

(III) *Open reduction.* This is used only after failure of the above methods. It may, however, be the first choice in fractures that will require internal fixation, such as displaced intra-articular fractures (referred to as open reduction and internal fixation, or ORIF). It has the advantage of allowing an accurate reduction but carries the risks and complications of an operation.

(3) **Restriction**

Once the fracture is reduced, it must be held in that position to allow the fracture to heal.

Some fractures are inherently *stable*, due to splintage from the adjacent soft tissues surrounding the fracture. These fractures tend to stay in the reduced position. Logic suggests that you do not need to support these fractures, although in practice they are often splinted (for example in a plaster cast) because of the risk that they may be knocked and may displace again (and also to reduce the pain and rest the affected part). Other fractures that are liable to displace after having been reduced are called *unstable* fractures, and these need to be kept in position by other methods.

Methods of Restriction

(I)   *Nonrigid methods of support.* Slings and elastic supports.

(II)   *Plaster fixation.* The commonest is plaster of paris. Newer plasters are lighter and stronger, although more expensive. All plasters can soften if they become wet, and the position can be lost. Either a back slab is used initially or a full cast is applied which is split longitudinally to accommodate any early swelling and prevent compartment syndrome (see later). The plaster is then *completed* by application of a full plaster after one or two days as the swelling subsides.

(III) *Functional bracing.* Here the joints are left free to move, but the shafts of the bone are supported in cast segments usually joined by hinges to allow movement only in one plane. This is most widely used for femoral or tibial fractures. As it is not all that strong, it is usual to wait until the fracture has begun to unite. So these fractures tend to be placed into a plaster cast for six weeks and are then converted to a functional brace. In the elderly with periarticular injuries, functional bracing can be the first line of treatment.

(IV)   *Continuous traction.* This is skin or skeletal traction and can be maintained for several weeks. In adults it does not tend to be used much nowadays, due to the problems of prolonged bed rest and also for social and economic reasons. One common example of traction used nowadays to immobilize a fracture is the collar and cuff for certain shoulder fractures. Here the weight of the arm is used as the force of distraction.

(V) *External fixation.* The bony fragments are held in position by pins inserted through the skin and into the bone. The pins are held in position by an external mechanical support. This method is especially useful in the management of open fractures where internal fixation with permanent metalwork may in some cases be inadvisable due to the higher risk of infection. Although an ex-fix can also get infected, the pins can be removed more easily.

(VI) *Internal fixation.* Pins, plates, screws or large intramedullary nails are used to hold the bony fragments in position. They are usually left in permanently, although they can be removed if necessary once the fracture has united. Sometimes a bone graft (usually taken from the iliac crest) is used to aid fracture healing, especially if there are large areas of bone loss. The bone graft has no structural integrity and only acts as a framework on which new bone grows. Internal fixation is used when the reduction needs to be as near perfect as possible (such as when a joint surface is involved), and also in the management of certain fractures to aid early mobility of the patient (e.g. hip fractures) or where it will not be possible to maintain an acceptable position by splintage or traction alone (very unstable fractures). Internal fixation is often advocated in the management of multiply injured patients involving the lower extremity (especially femoral fractures), where early fixation has been shown to reduce complications such as fat embolism and respiratory distress syndrome.

(4) Rehabilitation

Just because one part of the body is injured does not mean that the patient has to stay in bed and rest. The remaining limbs should be mobilized to avoid other complications. The rehabilitation of the affected part really depends on what the fracture is. For example, after a hip operation most feel that it is important to get the patient up mobilising as soon as possible. The physiotherapists are involved early and help with exercises and mobility. Rehabilitation involves restoring not only the injured part, but also the patient as a whole. This means the occupational therapist should help with various splints, mobility aids and home modifications, the social services should be involved to increase resources such as home helps and meals on wheels, etc.

Listed above are all of the *options* for the management of fractures; you will, however, find that two surgeons at different hospitals may differ markedly in the way they treat the same fracture. This is because the decision on how a fracture should be treated depends on many factors, including:

- The nature of the accident and the complexity of the fracture
- The condition of the skin and soft tissues
- Any associated injuries
- The age and general health of the patient
- The facilities available
- The skill of the surgeon

COMPLICATIONS OF FRACTURES

General Complications

Complications of Any Tissue Damage

- Haemorrhage and shock
- Fat embolism and respiratory distress syndrome
- Infection
- Muscle damage and rhabdomyolysis

Complications of Prolonged Bed Rest

- Chest infection and urinary tract infection
- Pressure sores and muscle wasting
- Deep vein thrombosis and pulmonary embolus

Complications of Anaesthesia (see Chap. 4)

Complications Specific to the Fracture

Immediate	Haemorrhage
	Neurovascular and visceral damage
Early	Compartment syndrome
	Infection
Late	Problems with union (delayed, non- and malunion)
	Avascular necrosis
	Sudek's atrophy
	Myositis ossificans
	Joint stiffness
	Growth disturbance

Compartment Syndrome

In the limbs there are osteofascial compartments. The muscles are divided into separate compartments by membranes that join the bone to the subcutaneous fascia. Swelling that occurs after a fracture can lead to an increase in the pressure within one of these compartments. The capillary blood flow to the tissues becomes reduced, leading to ischaemia. After about six hours irreversible changes begin to occur and muscle and nerve necrosis results. The muscle once infarcted is replaced by fibrous tissue which will lead to contractures (Volkman's ischaemic contracture). The same process can occur in a limb that is inside a plaster that is too tight. The patients classically have pain that is out of proportion to clinical findings. The six P's of acute ischaemia should be looked for, namely

Pain, Pallor, Paraesthesia, a Perishingly cold limb and later on Pulselessness and Paralysis. However, the best and earliest sign of compartment syndrome is pain on passive stretching of the muscles of the affected compartment (for the forearm flexor compartment this means stretching the fingers straight). If you wait until the pulses have disappeared, it will be too late anyway. The common sites for compartment syndrome are the forearm and the lower limb (especially with tibial fractures).

If you are called to see a patient in whom you suspect compartment syndrome, your initial management is to elevate the limb, remove all of the bandages and split the cast (if not split already); if this fails to relieve the pain, then you should remove the plaster. Ask a senior immediately to assess the patient. It is possible to measure the compartment pressures directly, using probes if facilities allow. Treatment involves performing a fasciotomy to relieve the pressure.

Neurological Complications

Actual nerve severance is rare, but stretching over a bony edge in a fracture or dislocation is more common. Examples of nerve palsies include axillary nerve palsy (dislocation of the shoulder), radial nerve palsy (fracture of the shaft of the humerus), ulnar nerve palsy (elbow dislocation), sciatic nerve palsy (dislocated hip) and common peroneal nerve palsy (fracture of the neck of the fibula or knee dislocation). Nerve palsies are usually reversible, although it can sometimes take months before the function returns to normal.

Problems with Union

Delayed union vs nonunion

There is no exact time that a fracture should take to heal, but some fractures take longer than would be expected (for a person of that age), and this is called delayed union. If the bone fails to unite, then the fracture eventually goes on to a state of nonunion. There is no exact distinction in terms of the time when you should call it delayed as opposed to nonunion; however, if the bone has failed to unite after several months, it is unlikely to heal without intervention and is described as nonunion.

The cause of delayed union and nonunion is unknown but, undoubtedly, poor blood supply, excessive shearing forces between the fragments, infection, interposition of tissue between the fragments, etc., all contribute.

Nonunion has two characteristic X-ray appearances. Usually the bone ends look rounded (like elephant feet) and appear dense and sclerotic, and this is called *hypertrophic nonunion*. In some cases a false joint may form (pseudoarthrosis) between the two ends. In these cases there is plenty of new bone formation but for some reason the two ends do not unite (perhaps because of movement or interposed tissues). Less commonly, the bone can look osteopenic, and it is then called *atrophic nonunion*, which is probably due to inadequate blood supply.

In the case of a nonunion the patient may require an operation such as ORIF and/or bone grafting to help the fracture unite (bone morphogenic protein, or BMP, is another substance being studied to act as a promoter of bone formation, but only as a research tool at present).

Malunion

This is where the fracture has healed in an imperfect position, either shortened, angulated or rotated. It may cause an unsightly appearance despite good function, or it may look fine but functionally have a poor result (especially if a joint is involved). Worse still, it may be both.

Avascular Necrosis

Avascular necrosis (AVN) is the death of part of a bone due to a deficient blood supply. Common sites for this to occur include the head of the femur, the scaphoid and the talus after fractures or dislocations where the blood supply is disrupted. The affected bones become soft and deformed, causing pain, stiffness and osteoarthritis. X-ray changes include sclerosis of the affected bone, which may appear distorted in shape; however, symptoms usually appear before any radiological changes.

Sudek's Atrophy (Post-traumatic Osteodystrophy)

This is a condition where the patient suffers chronic pain in the affected limb. It is usually not noticed until the plaster has been removed, several weeks after the injury. There may be associated swelling of the limb. For example, in a small proportion of patients following a Colles' fracture there can be swelling of the hands and fingers, the skin is warm, pink and glazed in appearance, movement is decreased, and the wrist and hand are painful to touch. It can also be seen in the lower limb. The cause is thought to be due to autonomic changes with an unusual sympathetic response. Although the condition is usually self-limiting, some patients find it disabling and are under the care of pain specialists. Guanethidine nerve blocks and sympathectomy seem to help in some cases.

Myositis Ossificans (Post-traumatic Ossification)

This is a condition where calcification forms in the soft tissues around a joint, causing restricted, painful movement. The commonest site for this is the elbow region. The exact cause is unknown but thought to be due to calcification and then ossification of blood that collected during the trauma. The affected area may be excised surgically at a later date if necessary.

Growth Disturbance

Children's injuries at the epiphyseal end of long bones can be categorized according to the Salter–Harris Classification.

X-rays in children are difficult to interpret, as the growth plate is often

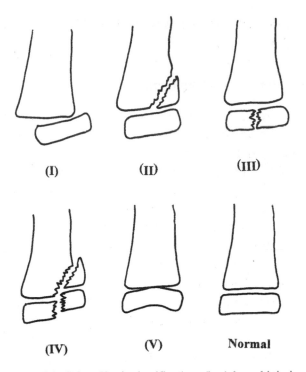

Figure 15.4. Salter–Harris classification of epiphyseal injuries.

confused for a fracture. If there is damage to the growth plate (also called physis), abnormal growth may result. If a fracture goes through the epiphyseal plate (e.g. Salter–Harris I), provided good reduction is achieved there may be normal growth. Small amounts of displacement are often acceptable in children's fractures, since they tend to remodel (especially in the plane of movement) as the child grows. The worst fractures are the ones where a growth plate injury, such as a crush, is missed at the time of the injury (e.g. Salter–Harris V) and are not picked up until growth is distorted. Many fractures in children can be treated by manipulation under anaesthetic and then immobilization in plaster. Intra-articular epiphyseal injuries are usually treated by ORIF.

FRACTURES YOU SHOULD KNOW SOMETHING ABOUT FOR FINALS

Fractures of the Neck of the Femur

Some like to refer to this group as fractures of the proximal femur. They occur mainly in elderly females, usually with osteoporotic bone, and are therefore by definition pathological fractures. There is usually a history of a fall with the patient being unable to get up afterwards (in some cases the fracture may occur spontaneously and precede the fall). These fractures have a high mortality (up to 40% at one year) no matter what treatment is performed in the initial period. The exact reason for this high mortality is unclear (even if you take into account the age and coexisting medical problems) and is studied all the time.

If the patient has a history of a fall and clinical findings support the diagnosis of a fractured neck of the femur but the X-rays appear normal, then a bone scan can be performed, which may show a hot spot at the fracture site.

The normal finding on examination is to see the leg lying externally rotated and shortened (due to the pull of iliopsoas on the femoral shaft, which is now independent of the hip joint). All movements may be painful and they usually cannot bear weight.

When clerking the patient you should pay particular attention to her social circumstances. You need to document what her mobility had been like prior to the fall (did she walk independently or did she need a stick or frame, etc.?), does she live alone, in a warden-controlled flat or in a nursing home? How many floors and stairs does her house have and who does her shopping, cleaning and cooking? You should also document the patient's mini-mental-test score. In general the prognosis is better if she was cognitively intact, mobile and independent previously. This also gives you a guide as to what she will be likely to achieve afterwards.

These fractures are classified as intra- or extracapsular, depending on whether the fracture is proximal or distal to the capsular insertion (which is along the intertrochanteric line). You may recall that the main

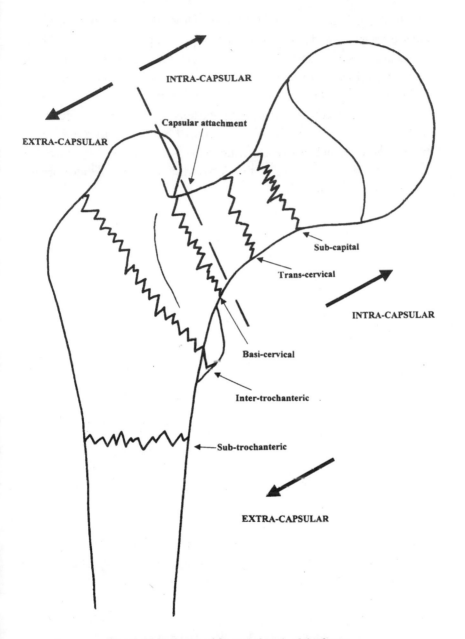

Figure 15.5. Types of fractured neck of the femur.

blood supply to the head of the femur comes from vessels that travel under the capsule and along the neck (a small supply is also derived from nutrient vessels in the shaft and from a vessel that travels in the ligamentum teres). Therefore, if a fracture is intracapsular then the blood supply to the head is compromised. It is impossible to tell which fractures will go on to develop avascular necrosis, but logic tells you that the more displaced the head is, the more likely the vessels will have been torn and hence there is more chance of avascular necrosis. Extracapsular fractures, on the other hand, usually have an intact blood supply and are therefore not at risk of avascular necrosis.

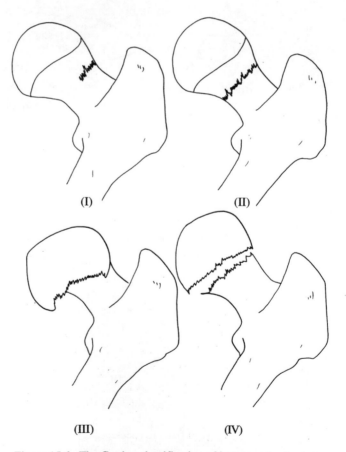

Figure 15.6. The Garden classification of intracapsular fractures.

Intracapsular Fractures

Intracapsular fractures are described as subcapital or transcervical, and are grouped into four types according to the Garden classification (Garden I–IV). Garden I and II are undisplaced and Garden III and IV are displaced.

Undisplaced intracapsular fractures are often impacted and would unite if left alone, although the aim nowadays should be to mobilize such patients as soon as possible to avoid the complications of prolonged bed rest and reduce the load on long term hospital beds. Also, about 30% will go on to displace if not fixed. The fracture is therefore stabilized at operation, usually by the insertion of parallel screws through the neck and into the head to hold it in position.

Displaced intracapsular fractures will not usually unite without reduction. Because of the disrupted blood supply to the head of the femur, many of such patients go on to develop avascular necrosis (AVN). An operation could be performed to reduce the fracture and hold it in position with screws; however, if you follow the patients up over the next few months many of them will still have pain and require a second operation (due to AVN of the femoral head). For this reason, in the elderly many surgeons would recommend excising the femoral head and replacing it with a prosthesis (hemiarthroplasty, or half-a-hip replacement) at the initial operation. There are many types of prostheses available. In the Thompson or Austin–Moore prostheses the false head articulates with the acetabulum. The Austin–Moore is an uncemented prosthesis and the Thompson is cemented.

In the young patient (aged less than 65) you need to consider the long term outcome. The disruption to the blood supply is dependent on the severity of the initial trauma, but early reduction may prevent subsequent AVN. A hip replacement lasts only 10–20 years and thus you may want to try to preserve the patient's own joint for as long as possible. Therefore, all intracapsular fractures in the young should be booked for theatre as an emergency and undergo reduction and have internal fixation (usually with screws). Young patients should be followed up in the outpatient clinic, and if they continue to have pain they can have a total hip replacement at a later date.

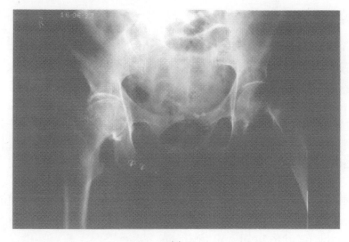

(a)

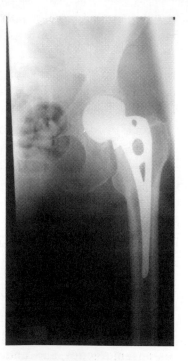

(b)

Figure 15.7. (a) Displaced intracapsular fractured neck of the femur (left); (b) Austin–Moore hemiarthroplasty (left).

Extracapsular Fractures

Extracapsular fractures can be described as basicervical, intertrochanteric or subtrochanteric, depending on the relationship to the trochanters, and they do not carry the same risk of avascular necrosis. They can be managed nonoperatively but again most orthopaedic surgeons advocate early mobilization and hence we tend to fix these fractures. Fixing these fractures also helps reduce the amount of pain. The commonest operation nowadays for these fractures is the insertion of a dynamic hip screw (DHS). In this procedure the patient is placed on the fracture table and the foot is placed into a traction boot. A closed reduction is performed (traction is applied to the leg to reduce the fracture, under image intensifier control). An incision is made over the greater trochanter and a screw is inserted into the femoral head under image intensifier control. A plate attaches to the DHS and rests along the shaft of the femur, to which it is fixed by screws. The angle between the plate and the screw is 135°, which is the usual angle between the neck and the shaft in most people. The screw is "dynamic", because it can move slightly in relation to the plate. These fractures have a natural tendency to collapse and so the screw can slide along the plate to accommodate this. It will not, however, allow rotational movements.

In summary, get a good history, site a venflon, send off U&E's, FBC and a group and save and get an ECG and a chest X-ray. If necessary, correct the patient's medical problems (she is usually dehydrated and requires fluid resuscitation), optimizing her for theatre. If the patient is in severe discomfort skin traction can be applied to reduce the pain. Extracapsular fractures are reduced and internally fixed (usually a DHS). Intracapsular fractures, if nondisplaced, undergo fixation (screws) and, if displaced, undergo a hemiarthroplasty. There is a saying commonly used by medical students that applies to intracapsular fractures classified by Garden: "One, two, screw, three, four Austin–Moore." Remember that this applies to patients over 65. All young patients with intracapsular fractures should be booked as an emergency and the fractures should be accurately reduced and internally fixed.

Postoperatively the patients should be examined to ensure that they are comfortable and that there is no evidence of a neurovascular deficit,

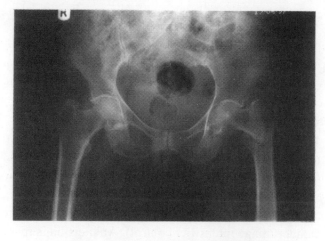

(a)

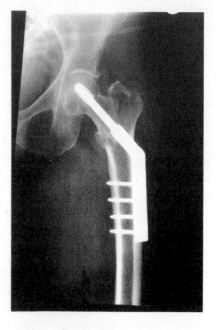

(b)

Figure 15.8. (a) Extracapsular fractured neck of the femur (left); (b) dynamic hip screw (DHS) fixation (left).

and they should have a check full blood count and X-ray. Provided the X-rays are satisfactory they are usually mobilized after a day or two by the physiotherapists.

Radius and Ulna Shaft

Isolated fractures of either of these bones are uncommon, and if they are seen one should suspect an associated dislocation at either the proximal or the distal radioulnar joint. These fracture dislocations are known by their Italian eponyms. A fracture of the ulna shaft with dislocation of the radial head is called a Monteggia fracture (the radial head should normally lie in front of the capitellum). A Galleazzi fracture is a fracture of the radial shaft with a dislocation of the distal (or inferior) radioulnar joint.

These fractures are unstable and are usually treated by ORIF in adults. In children the fracture is usually manipulated under anaesthetic (if manipulation is required) and treated in plaster.

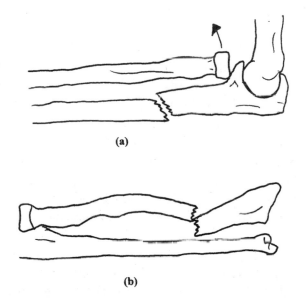

(a)

(b)

Figure 15.9. Types of forearm fractures: (a) Monteggia fracture; (b) Galeazzi fracture.

If a fracture of the forearm is being treated in plaster, then it should be left in the most stable position. Fractures of the proximal radius and ulna are said to be most stable in supination, distal fractures are said to be most stable in pronation, and fractures of the mid-shaft are said to be most stable in neutral. For example, a mid-shaft radial fracture is plastered with the hand in neutral (mid-pronation). The plaster is extended above the elbow to prevent any supination or pronation.

Fractures of the Distal Radius

Fractures of the distal radius have for some reason been associated with their eponymous names more than any other type of fracture. They can be classified in many ways, although the most commonly observed fracture is that which was described by an Irishman called Abraham Colles in 1814, long before the invention of radiography. He observed a deformity of the wrist similar in shape to a dinner fork, and hence called that a "dinner fork" deformity, usually in an elderly patient after a fall on to an outstretched hand. He described an extra-articular fracture of the distal radius (within an inch and a half of the joint) with dorsal displacement and radial shift of the distal fragment, and because the fragments are impacted there is also radial shortening (in addition, the ulna styloid is often pulled off by the triangular articular disc).

On examination, as with any fracture, the neurovascular function should be documented as the median nerve and the radial artery lie close. If the fracture is displaced, then treatment involves correction of the deformity and this is usually by manipulation. This can be performed under regional anaesthetic, e.g. Bier's block.

The reduction aims to improve two things: (1) restore the length (the articular surface of the distal radius should be more distal than the ulna), and (2) correct the angulation to allow for optimum function and minimal deformity.

The wrist is manipulated in the direction opposite to the forces which caused it in the first place, and therefore it should be flexed slightly with some ulna deviation (with the forearm fully pronated). A Colles plaster is applied from the elbow to the metarcarpophalangeal joints, and it encompasses the thumb metarcarpal, again leaving the thumb phalanges free to move. The plaster is usually split for a day or so and then completed when the swelling has subsided (an alternative is to place a back slab on initially, which is completed after a few days).

The position of the fracture should always be rechecked once in plaster to see if it has moved. If the position is still unacceptable or the fragments redisplace or the injury is intra-articular, then surgery may be required either as a external fixator, K wires or ORIF with plates and screws.

If treated in plaster this usually remains on for five or six weeks; meanwhile movement at the fingers, elbow and shoulder should be encouraged. Once the plaster is removed the wrist will need rehabilitation exercises by the physiotherapists.

The complications of a Colles fracture are commonly asked about in finals. The specific complications are malunion, median nerve problems (usually in badly reduced fractures), a stiff "frozen" shoulder (due to immobilisation), tendon rupture (the tendon of the extensor pollicis longus rubs along the distal radial fragment and often ruptures several weeks after the fracture) and, rarely, Sudek's atrophy.

Other injuries that can be caused by a fall on to an outstretched hand include fractures or dislocations of the phalanges, scaphoid fractures, radial and ulnar fractures, elbow dislocation or fracture, humeral shaft fracture, shoulder dislocation, rotator cuff tears and shoulder girdle injuries (subluxation of acromioclavicular joint, clavicular fracture, etc.).

A *Smith's fracture* is also called a "reverse Colles" and is usually caused by a fall on to the back of a flexed wrist. The distal radial fragment is displaced anteriorly. The fracture can be manipulated and placed into an above elbow cast with the wrist slightly extended and the forearm pronated. These fractures are very unstable and the fragments often slip. Close follow-up is therefore needed, with regular X-rays, and if the position slips, ORIF may be required

A *Barton's fracture* is the eponym used for a fracture dislocation where the distal radial fracture is oblique and extends into the wrist joint. You probably just need to have heard of it for the sake of finals.

Scaphoid Fractures

Diagnosis of a scaphoid fracture is often made from the history and the finding of tenderness in the anatomical snuffbox. Special "scaphoid" X-ray views should be requested when this injury is suspected. Often the X-ray appearance is normal until about 10 days after the injury. Therefore, if you suspect a scaphoid fracture you are obliged to treat it even with a normal X-ray. The wrist is placed in a scaphoid plaster which includes the thumb (the hand is in a beer-glass-holding position). The patient is advised to return to the fracture clinic after 10 days for a re-X-ray. The fracture may now become apparent due to local decalcification. If the patient is nontender and X-rays are normal, the plaster can be removed and the patient discharged. If the X-ray is still normal but the patient is still tender, then the plaster should really be replaced for a further two weeks. A bone scan may sometimes be helpful in making the diagnosis.

The main concern with this fracture is the risk of avascular necrosis. The blood supply to the scaphoid is via small vessels that enter the bone distally and hence the proximal fragment is at risk of becoming avascular (especially if displaced), leaving the patient with pain and stiffness in the wrist.

Scaphoid fractures require a plaster for six weeks, after which time the wrist is reassessed by X-rays and clinical examination. If a complication such as delayed union or nonunion occurs, then either the arm can be placed in a plaster for a further six weeks or ORIF and bone grafting may be considered.

Supracondylar Fractures of the Humerus

These injuries are most common in children, usually after a fall on to an outstretched hand. The elbow is very swollen and is held in a semiflexed position.

The distal fragment usually displaces backwards and the sharp edge of the proximal humerus may compress or injure the brachial artery which lies close to it. The child needs to be admitted and have the fracture

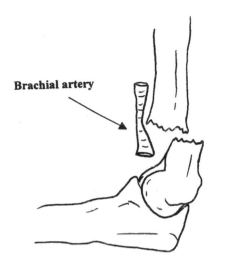

Brachial artery

Figure 15.10. Supracondylar fracture of the humerus.

manipulated under anaesthesia with image intensifier control. If satisfactory reduction is obtained, the arm can be placed in an above elbow backslab or a collar and cuff (obviously ensuring that there is a good radial pulse). If the fracture is very unstable, then fixation with pins or wires may be required. Because of the risk of compartment syndrome, the child needs to be observed very carefully over the next 24 h. Pain on passive extension (stretching the flexor compartment) of the fingers is the earliest warning sign of compartment syndrome. The elbow should be extended slightly to see if this restores the circulation, but if this fails surgical exploration of the radial artery is needed, otherwise Volkmann's ischaemic contracture can result. This is where the forearm muscles become fibrosed and shortened, leading to a "claw hand" deformity.

Dislocated Shoulder

Almost all such cases are anterior dislocations (95%). Because the shoulder is the most mobile of all the joints, its stability is sacrificed, especially inferiorly where the rotator cuff is deficient.

Dislocation is usually caused by direct trauma or falling on to the hand. The humeral head is driven forwards, tearing the capsule and sometimes the glenoid labrum as well. There may be an associated fracture of the greater tuberosity of the humerus.

The patient is in severe pain reluctant to any examination of the shoulder. The normal curved contour of the shoulder may be lost and may appear square. The arm is supported by the opposite hand.

It is vital that you examine for any distal neurovascular deficit, especially of the axillary nerve, which can be damaged during the dislocation. The axillary nerve supplies a small egg-shaped patch of skin over the insertion of the deltoid and should be tested both before and after reduction (the axillary nerve also supplies the deltoid but the muscle can obviously not be examined whilst the shoulder is dislocated).

X-rays should be an AP and an axillary lateral view to see in which direction the humeral head has gone in relation to the glenoid.

Reduction is usually performed under sedation in the casualty department. One method has the patient in the supine position with the arm abducted, and an assistant applies countertraction to the body (maybe with a towel held around the patient's chest under the axilla). The head can be guided back into the socket by a third assistant. An alternative is to have the patient prone with the arm hanging and some weights attached to it for traction. (Kocher's method is not recommended, as it can cause a fracture of the greater tuberosity). If these methods fail then reduction may be attempted under general anaesthetic. The arm can then be rested in a sling (to avoid external rotation) for about 3–4 weeks.

Posterior dislocation of the shoulder is easily overlooked (and occasionally you will see a patient who sustained a posterior dislocation several days or weeks prior that had been missed). It is caused by direct trauma (and is seen in epileptics). The AP X-ray may give the impression of the humeral head sitting in the glenoid (hence it is missed), although it may appear rounded — the so-called "light bulb" sign (due to internal rotation, and hence the greater tuberosity is not seen).

Femoral and Tibial Fractures

In these injuries, resuscitate the patient and deal with life-threatening injuries first. Blood loss can be great, so cross-match two units in tibial fractures and four units in femoral fractures. A traction splint can be applied for femoral fractures, and a padded board or long leg splint can be used for tibial fractures. Both are at risk of compartment syndrome. In the young most of these fractures are treated surgically. The state-of-the-art treatment for femoral or tibial fractures is to use an intramedullary nail (a long nail placed right down the centre from the top end to hold the fracture). There are alternative treatments, including a plate and screws or an external fixator. Each method has advantages and disadvantages (for example, the pins of an external fixator go through the muscles in the thigh-limiting rehabilitation), and for the sake of finals you need to know that all are acceptable options. If the fracture is "open", management is different (see above), antibiotics are started, and the patient is taken to theatre for debridement and washout. The fracture is then assessed and stabilized (usually with an intramedullary nail for the femur and an external fixator or intramedullary nail for tibial fractures).

There have been studies showing that patients who have their femoral fractures stabilised within 24 h do better in terms of respiratory complications (e.g. chest infection and ARDS) than patients who are left for longer before the operation. One of the main factors in this is that nursing care is made easier, allowing the patients to be sat up once they have been fixed.

Knee Injuries

Sportsmen are very prone to knee injuries, in which several structures can be damaged. The collateral ligaments get torn in valgus or varus strains. Twisting injuries can lead to meniscal tears or a rupture of the anterior cruciate ligament (ACL). There is a triad which can occur often in a sporting rotational injury where the anterior cruciate, the medial meniscus and the medial collateral ligament are torn ("the unhappy triad of O'Donoghue").

In the history you must ask whether the knee swelled up immediately or overnight. If the knee swells immediately, this points to a haemarthrosis, which often occurs with fractures or torn cruciates. Overnight swelling indicates an effusion, which may in turn imply a meniscal tear or another ligamentous injury.

When the patient presents immediately after the injury, this is all you can ask about and examination essentially is limited to noting an effusion and any areas of tenderness. Testing for menisci or cruciate damage when the knee is acutely swollen is difficult. An X-ray should be taken to ensure there are no fractures, and initially the treatment is Rest, Ice packs, Compression or splintage, and Elevation (RICE). Once the swelling has subsided the knee can be re-examined for meniscal or cruciate damage.

If the patient presents some time after the injury, then the history usually points to the diagnosis. Symptoms that you should ask about include pain, locking, swelling and giving way. Locking means that the patient cannot fully extend the knee because of a mechanical obstruction, such as a meniscal tear. Giving way is usually a sign of instability, such as a torn anterior cruciate ligament, but may occur because of pain. A history of locking, together with the finding of an effusion and joint line tenderness, usually indicates a meniscal tear.

If a meniscal tear or torn cruciate is suspected, then an arthroscopy can be performed (an MRI can be used for diagnosis but is expensive and does not allow anything to be done).

An arthroscopy means the knee is looked into with a camera. The knee is first re-examined under anaesthesia and then an arthroscope is inserted into it and the three joint compartments are inspected — the patellofemoral joint and the medial and lateral compartments. If a meniscal tear is seen it can be excised and trimmed using various instruments and shavers. The outer third of the meniscus is the only part that has any blood supply and tears of this region are usually repaired if possible, since removal of the menisci predisposes to osteoarthritis. There are many types of meniscal tears, an example being a "bucket handle" tear, where the "bucket handle" can flip in and out of the joint space, causing locking. The cruciate ligaments are inspected and any tears are noted. The joint is washed out to clear any debris.

Postoperatively, early mobilization is encouraged, if necessary with the use of crutches until the pain subsides.

If a tear of the anterior cruciate ligament is noted, a reconstruction may be advised at a later date, after physiotherapy has been tried. In some people with a torn ACL there are other structures that give stability to the joint and you can strengthen the leg muscles sufficiently to avoid the need for reconstruction, although they may no longer be able to engage in activities that require very stable knees (for example playing football or going skiing). The patient's occupation is important, since a torn cruciate may not be as important in a person who works behind a desk as it is in a roofer who climbs up ladders. The reconstruction usually involves taking a graft from the hamstrings or the patella tendon and rerouting it through the knee. Postoperatively movement is encouraged early on and a vigorous physiotherapy rehabilitation programme is commenced. It takes many months and lots of hard work to restore the patient to near normal function.

OSTEOARTHRITIS

Osteoarthritis (OA) is a very common disorder, and it is likely that there will be a finals long case involving this disease and so it is covered in some detail. It is a degenerative joint disorder in which there is progressive loss of articular cartilage. OA can be *primary*, where there is no obvious underlying cause, or *secondary*, when it follows a pre-existing abnormality of the joint (e.g. fracture, rheumatoid disease, haemarthrosis, meniscal tear, etc).

All normal articular surfaces are lined by a thin layer of hyaline cartilage (in the knee there is an additional "shock absorber" — the menisci, which are made of fibrocartilage). Initially there is softening of the articular cartilage and the normally smooth surface becomes frayed (or fibrillated), fissured, and eventually is worn away to expose the underlying bone. The subchondral bone, which is now under greater stresses, becomes thickened and sclerotic, and cysts may form (due to microfractures). As the disease progresses the cartilage left in unstressed areas proliferates and ossifies to form bony outgrowths called osteophytes (which some would say are an attempt by the body to restabilise the joint). Capsular fibrosis may occur secondarily, leading to a stiff joint. All synovial joints may be affected, although the weight-bearing joints, such as the knee and the hip, tend to be the most common. If the spine is affected, then this is known as spondylosis (which may have complications, such as nerve root compression by osteophytes).

The exact aetiology of the disease is unknown and lots of work is being performed in this area. However, it is known that the frequency increases with age. We tend to think of OA as wear and tear, and this is how we explain it to our patients, but if it was simply wear and tear then everyone should suffer from symptomatic arthritis as they get older, but they do not. It presumably is multifactorial and involves not only the stresses that the cartilage is put under but also the ability of the cartilage to withstand the stresses.

Do not confuse osteoarthritis with osteoporosis or osteomalacia, which are completely different conditions. Osteoporosis is where the amount of bone stock is less than you should have and osteomalacia is where there is failure of mineralization (not enough calcification of the bone).

Symptoms

(1) *Pain.* This is the predominant symptom, usually aggravated by exercise and relieved by rest. It is progressive over months to years and there are often periods of remission and flare-ups, often due to trauma (the capsule may be stretched and inflamed). As the disease progresses and its severity worsens, the patient may have pain at night interfering with sleep.

(2) *Stiffness.* This occurs especially after long periods of rest, and hence the patient can be very stiff in the morning, but this tends to improve as the day goes on.

(3) *Deformity.* This is a feature of advanced disease and may result from muscular spasm, capsular and ligamentous contracture and distortion of the joint surface.

If you have a long case you should spend some time finding out about mobility, home circumstances, social services, family backup, etc. On examination movement is restricted, usually with accompanied crepitus, and in later stages of the disease there may be fixed flexion deformities. In the hands swellings may form at the distal interphalangeal joints known as Heberden's nodes, and if seen at the PIPJ's these are called Bouchard's nodes.

X-Ray Changes (Figure 15.11)

OA has the following X-ray changes:

(1) Narrowing of the joint space (as the cartilage is worn away) is the most important sign.
(2) Osteophytes — bits of bone overgrowth, usually near the edge of the joint
(3) Subchondral sclerosis.
(4) Subchondral bone cysts.
(5) There may be evidence of previous disorders, such as old fractures, rheumatoid or congenital defects.

Management

In the early stages of the disease, treatment is conservative, using analgesics, weight loss, advice on altering load-bearing activities such as increased periods of rest, use of walking sticks or avoidance of activities that exacerbate the condition (in the younger patient this may mean giving up his sport or changing his job). Physiotherapy to help increase the joint mobility and strengthen the muscles is often of great help. Injection of steroids and local anaesthetic into the joint space during acute flare-ups may be of some benefit.

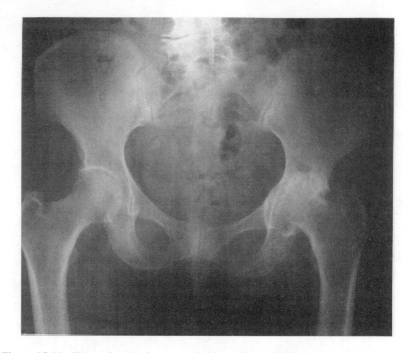

Figure 15.11. X-ray changes in osteoarthritis — the right hip has some osteoarthritic changes, although compared to the left hip it has relatively well-preserved joint space. On the left the joint space is completely obliterated; there are bone cysts, subchondral sclerosis and osteophytes. See Figure 15.12 for the postop film.

Patients often cope with their symptoms for many years. If, however, symptoms progress despite all of the above measures, then the following surgical options are available:

Arthroscopic washout. The commonest site for this is the knee, and the severity of the disease is assessed directly (and graded I–IV). The frayed cartilage is trimmed and any loose bodies are removed (pieces of cartilage or broken-off osteophytes). The joint is washed out to remove any remaining debris, and local anaesthetic is injected (sometimes a partial synovectomy is performed).

Osteotomy. This means the bone is divided, and sometimes a small area of the bone is removed to correct the deformity. Once divided the bone is left to unite either by external plaster or by internal fixation. Osteotomy can help relieve the pain but why it works is unknown (it is thought that it may be due to adjustment of the weight-bearing surfaces and changes in blood flow to the bone).

Arthrodesis. This means the joint is fused and will therefore restrict mobility. It is mainly used as a last resort for joints where the loss of movement is not too disabling (for example in the toes). For the hip and the knee, fusion is rarely performed nowadays unless infection is a complication.

Arthroplasty. This can be replacement or excisional arthroplasty. In some joints, such as the metartarsophalangeal joints of the foot, it is better to excise the arthritic joint, allowing a fibrous and pain-free joint to form in its place. The hip and the knee have received the most attention for replacement arthroplasty, although there are many other prostheses available for the shoulder, the elbow and almost any other joint (although results have been poor in many joints, such as the ankle). The results for hip and knee replacements are so good that nowadays an osteotomy is less commonly performed and arthrodesis is rarely indicated initially. We try to avoid joint replacement in the young (less than age 65), as it may last only 10–20 years before needing revision and the results of revision surgery are not as good as those of primary surgery. Nowadays, however, some joint replacements are lasting longer and longer and are being used in younger age groups because the alternatives are nowhere near as good.

Total Hip Replacement

The total hip replacement (THR) was developed by Sir John Charnley in the 1960's and is now a very successful procedure for arthritis of the hip (with a good result in about 95% of cases). The worn acetabulum is replaced by a high density polyethylene cup into which a ceramic or metal head (part of the femoral stem) articulates. The components are usually cemented in place using an antibiotic-containing bone cement (although newer, uncemented prostheses are available which are coated or "sintered" and allow bone to grow into them; they are often used in younger patients, who are more likely to need revisions at a later date).

An incision (e.g. posterolateral) is made over the hip and the fascia lata needs to be divided to gain access to the capsule of the joint. The head of the femur is dislocated and then the wear or damage to the acetabulum and femur can be assessed. The head of the femur is removed, the acetabulum is prepared and the cup is cemented in (although uncemented prostheses are available). A hole is reamed (drilled) down the femoral shaft and, after a few trial stems are used, the correct prosthesis is cemented in (again, uncemented prostheses are available). The head is relocated into the acetabulum and the function of the joint

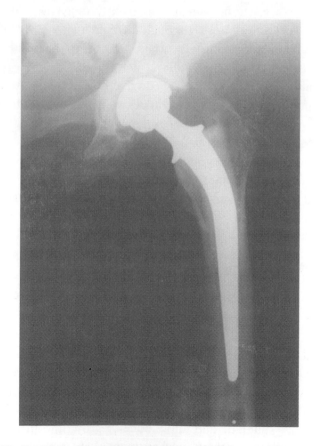

Figure 15.12. Total hip replacement — both the acetabulum and femoral head have been replaced (note the cement around the femoral stem).

is tested to see if it is stable. The soft tissues are closed in layers, with two or three drains usually needed (which stay in for 24–48 h). The leg is placed in slight abduction using a triangular pillow, to maintain good position of the joint.

Rehabilitation begins about a day or so after the operation, initially with leg exercises, and once the X-rays have been checked the patient is allowed to fully weight-bear. The usual hospital stay is about 7–12 days. If an uncemented prosthesis is used, then the patient remains partially weight-bearing with crutches for about six weeks (to allow the tissues to heal and bone to form around the prosthesis), after which time he can start to fully weight-bear.

About 85% of THR's last over 10 years. After about 10 years, up to 10% can loosen and may need revision. However, the success rate of revision hips is not as good as the primary operation. Complications include dislocation, and about 3% of primary THR's dislocate and the patients are therefore advised against squatting or sitting on low chairs or movements that adduct the hip (i.e. sit with their legs crossed), which can cause dislocation. Studies have shown that up to 50% of THR's suffer a DVT and the risk is approximately halved with heparin prophylaxis. The risk of a PE is about 1–2%. Joint infection (about 1%) is disastrous and will require revision (in many cases this is performed as a two-stage procedure where the metalwork is removed in order to clear the infection (a Girdlestone's procedure) and traction is applied for several weeks before a definitive revision can be performed.

Total Knee Replacement

The total knee replacement (TKR) came after the THR and the exact life expectancy is still not known, although some knee replacements have lasted over 20 years. Despite bad press in the past, the success rate of this operation is now excellent.

The joint is made of two metal prostheses with an intervening polyethylene articular disc between the distal femur and the tibial plateau. If only one compartment of the joint is damaged, this can be replaced by a unicompartmental prosthesis, although results of this have not been as encouraging.

The knee is fully flexed and a tourniquet is usually applied and the leg prepared. An incision is made in the mid-line (about 10 inches long). The joint is accessed via the medial side of the patella as the patella is flipped back laterally. The distal femur and the tibial plateau are prepared by sawing off the irregular surfaces to allow the prostheses to fit on (using special devices to ensure all the angles are correct). Trial prostheses are used to attain the correct sizes to allow for optimal function and stability

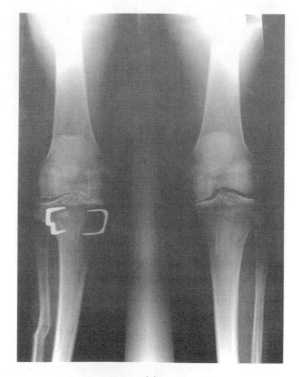

(a)

Figure 15.13. (a) Osteoarthritis of both knees — the medial compartment is more severely affected on both knees. Note that there are staples from an old right tibial osteotomy. (b) Right total knee replacement (TKR). AP view. (c) Lateral view (patellar surface has not been replaced).

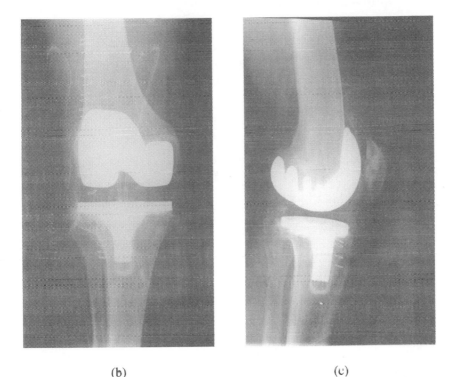

(b)   (c)

Figure 15.13 (*continued*)

of the joint. The prostheses are cemented into place (again, uncemented prostheses are available and are being compared in trials) and a polyethylene disc is inserted between the tibia and the femur, acting like the articular cartilage, ensuring there is no contact between the metal parts. The tibial component can have either a short or a long stem. The anterior cruciate ligament is divided and the posterior cruciate is sometimes kept. If the patella surface is worn, then it can also be replaced by a polyethylene prosthesis. The knee is washed out and the function is again tested, ensuring good flexion, patellar tracking and stability. Closure is again in layers, usually with two or three drains. A check X-ray is taken on day 2 or 3.

Postoperatively the leg is placed in to a splint for support and protection. Bending of the knee is begun after one or two days, and once active straight leg raising is achieved the patient can begin partial weight bearing, progressing to full weight bearing. The hospital stay is usually about 10 days and the patient should be mobilizing independently, achieving flexion to 90° with a good active straight leg raise before discharge.

Complications include DVT, which occurs in about 50–75% of TKR's (the incidence is halved if heparin prophylaxis is used), although many are asymptomatic. The risk of pulmonary embolus is about 1% (although fatal PE is said to be < 0.1%). The infection rate is about 3% and is a disaster because the success of revision knees is again much lower than that of the primary procedure.

RHEUMATOID ARTHRITIS

Rheumatoid arthritis (RA) is a large subject that usually comes up in the medical section of the exam; however, there are many operative procedures that can be performed to help the patients and you should know just a little about this. There are three goals in the treatment of RA:

(1) *Prevention and treatment of the inflammatory synovitis.* Advice, exercises, joint protection and drugs such as the disease-modifying drugs — gold, penecillamine and immunosuppressants.

(2) *Prevention of joint destruction and deformity.* Rest during acute exacerbations followed by rehabilitation and physiotherapy. RA patients are prone to tendon rupture, which may require operative repair.

(3) *Joint reconstruction.* Joint replacements have a place in RA patients. The hip, knee, shoulder and elbow are examples of joints which can be replaced in advanced destruction, deformity or instability. You must, however, treat the symptoms and not the X-ray appearances. Other operations that have a place are arthrodesis, osteotomy and synovectomy.

The X-ray changes of RA include soft tissue swelling, joint space narrowing and, later on, articular destruction and deformity.

AVASCULAR NECROSIS

This often comes up in multiple choice or short answer sections. It is due to a disruption of the blood supply, either due to interruption of arterial inflow, such as after a fracture (covered above), or if venous outflow is blocked, as in infiltrative disorders that block the venous sinusoids (e.g. Gaucher's disease). The causes include:

- Fracture/dislocation.
- Sickle cell disease (clumping of the RBC's leads to diminished capillary flow. There is a tendency for the infarcted areas of bone to become infected with unusual organisms such as salmonella.
- Decompression sickness (caisson disease).
- Gaucher's disease (a rare familial disorder of lipid metabolism).
- Drug-induced (especially corticosteroids).
- Idiopathic.

X-rays initially show no changes; however, after a few weeks reactive new bone forms in the adjacent living tissue, showing up as an increased area of density. Later on the necrotic bone crumbles and the outline may be distorted. Bone scans show the region as an area of increased uptake due to the vascular reaction in the adjacent bone. The symptoms are usually pain and stiffness.

Idiopathic Avascular Necrosis (Osteochondritis)

In the above list the term "idiopathic" appears really for want of a better term. There is a group of conditions called osteochondritides, which are areas of patchy avascular necrosis of bone causing pain and limitation of movement, usually in adolescents. They are usually called by the names of those who described them, and examples include avascular necrosis of the second metatarsal head (Freiberg's disease), the navicular (Kohler's disease), the lunate (Kienb- ch's disease) and the capitulum of the humerus (Panner's disease).

The cause is unknown. There are two subgroups (traction aphophysitis and osteochondritis dissecans), which still come under the heading "osteochondritides", but because they have explainable causes they are listed below separately. Note that they are not inflammatory conditions and so the "itis" is not strictly correct.

Traction Apophysitis

Repetitive pulling forces of a tendon may damage the apophysis to which it is attached. The commonest example is the pull of the quadriceps on the tibial tuberosity, called Osgood–Schlatter disease (two separate surgeons who described the condition in the same year, 1903), which presents as knee pain, usually in growing adolescents, and responds to rest. Another example is Sever's disease of the calcaneum, due to the pull from the Achilles tendon.

Osteochondritis Dissecans

A piece of bone and its overlying articular cartilage may fall (dissect) off and into the joint space due to repeated minor stresses. The commonest site is the knee, with pain, swelling and limitation of movement. X-rays may show a loose body or a crater on the articular surface of the medial femoral condyle of the femur from which the fragment has fallen off. Treatment is usually conservative and symptoms often resolve although an arthroscopy may be necessary.

BONE TUMOURS

This is not a common topic in finals, although you may be asked to write an essay or discuss this during a viva. Because there are so many types, students often learn them as a list and therefore do not know the relative importance of each type. In fact all are incredibly rare, and what you must know is that primary bone tumours need to be managed by a specialist centre. Secondaries to bone are much more common.

In order to help you learn about bone tumours we think it is helpful to have a basic understanding of the terms used to describe bones, which cannot be understood without a brief introduction to the development

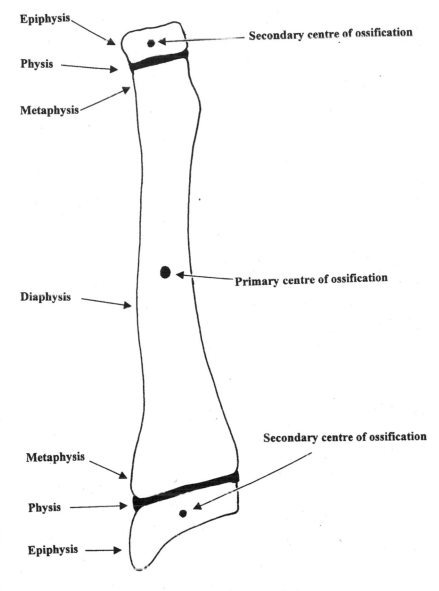

Figure 15.14. Development of a bone.

of long bones. A bone begins life as a cartilaginous model of approximately similar shape to the final product into which it will be converted.

The primary centre of ossification appears at the centre of the shaft or diaphysis (Greek for "in between") sometime during intrauterine life. The ossification spreads from here towards each end of the bone. Near the two ends of the bone there is a growth plate called the physis, from which longitudinal growth of the bone occurs initially as cartilage, which then undergoes ossification. At the outer end of the bone is the epiphysis (Greek for "on top") and this is also cartilaginous. Sometime after birth a secondary centre of ossification appears at each epiphyseal end. When you see an X-ray of a long bone of a child (depending on age), you see the ossified part of the epiphysis separated from the shaft by a gap, which is not actually a space but simply the unossified cartilaginous part of the bone. From the physis, bone is laid down towards the diaphysis into an area of bone called the metaphysis (Greek for "next to"). As the ossification from the primary centre and that from the secondary centre meet, fusion of the growth plate is said to occur, indicating skeletal maturity.

Primary bone tumours can develop in any of the tissues that make up the bone. They can be benign (given the ending "-oma") or malignant ("-sarcoma"). If derived from bone they are called osteoid tumours, such as an osteoma or osteosarcoma. Similarly, if they are derived from the cartilage they are called chondromas or chondrosarcomas, and if they are derived from the fibrous tissue they are called fibromas or fibrosarcoma. There are some tumours derived from the marrow, such as a Ewing's sarcoma or myeloma. Some of the benign tumours can become malignant.

Symptoms from bone tumours usually include pain and swelling, and certainly any such unexplained limb pain that lasts for more than a month (especially if pain occurs at night) should be investigated. The symptoms may be picked up incidentally on X-ray or present as a pathological fracture.

Most of the tumours have characteristic X-ray appearances; however, it is difficult to differentiate between benign and malignant tumours simply on this, and factors that suggest malignancy include rapid growth of a lesion, tenderness and warmth. If a malignancy is suspected, thorough investigation is needed to establish the exact diagnosis and assess the size and spread. Other investigations include a chest X-ray, bone scans, CT and MRI. The ESR is usually raised, as is the alkaline phosphatase. A biopsy should really be performed by the surgeon who will ultimately operate on the lesion, and therefore patients should be referred to a specialist centre early.

Primary Tumours

Osteoid osteomas. These are benign tumours that do not become malignant. They are small and usually occur in those under 30, most commonly in the tibia or femur. They appear on the X-ray as a small radiolucent area surrounded by dense sclerosis and are hot spots on a bone scan. The main symptom is pain which characteristically responds to aspirin. If left alone they may disappear spontaneously, but if the pain persists excision of the lesion can be undertaken, with instant resolution of the symptoms.

Osteochondromas. These are the commonest tumours of bone and are cartilage-capped exostoses which continue to grow as the bone grows (if multiple they may be part of a condition known as hereditary multiple exostoses). They usually present as a bony lump and appear on an X-ray as an abnormal outgrowth of bone — either finger-like or cauliflower-shaped projections (often they look smaller on an X-ray than they feel, as the cartilage does not show up). If there are symptoms they should be excised, and if they change in size after skeletal maturity, then this suggests possible malignancy (chondrosarcoma).

Chondromas and chondrosarcomas. Chondromas are benign tumours which can be single or multiple (Ollier's disease). They usually occur in the long bones (including the fingers). In patients over 30 it is important to exclude a chondrosarcoma, into which a chondroma can (rarely) develop. Chondrosarcomas usually affect the middle-aged to elderly age group and are found in the pelvis or the proximal end of the long bones. There are two types: one arises from the surface of the bone (sometimes in the cartilage-covered cap of an osteochondroma) and the other arises within the medulla of the bone, often as a chondroma that either becomes malignant or has in fact been a slow-growing malignancy all the time. X-rays show an expanding radiolucent lesion with characteristic flecks of calcification. Treatment is by excision or, if necessary, amputation, as chondrosarcomas tend to metastasise late. Five-year survival is about 50%.

Osteosarcomas. These occur in males more than in females, and usually in adolescents (although there is a second peak in those over 50, due to malignant change in Paget's disease). The commonest sites are around the knee or proximal humerus. Osteosarcomas usually occur in the metaphysis and are locally invasive, spreading distally via the blood (often to the lung). The main symptom is usually pain, especially at night, and there may be local tenderness. X-rays show a metaphyseal, translucent and destructive lesion. The tumour expands through the cortex, causing it to be raised, and a triangle of new bone is produced in the angle where the periosteum separates from the shaft called Codman's triangle. Eventually it breaks through the cortex into the surrounding soft tissues, causing streaks of calcification within them (the "sun-ray" appearance). Treatment usually involves chemotherapy and resection, which may mean amputation or wide local excision using an allograft or prostheses. About 60% survive five years.

Ewing's sarcomas. These are rare malignant tumours arising from the bone marrow, usually in young patients. Most of them occur in the diaphysis of long bones (in contrast to osteosarcomas). Again, they present with a painful swelling, although because the lump is usually warm and tender they are often diagnosed as having osteomyelitis. X-rays show a destructive lesion, sometimes with several layers of periosteal new bone around the lesion (called an "onion skin" appearance). Treatment is usually chemotherapy, followed by surgical excision if possible.

Giant cell tumours (osteoclastomas). These are of unknown origin, although there are multinuclear giant cells under the microscope, giving them their name. They occur in young adults, but only after fusion of the growth plate. They are usually around the knee (in the lower end of the femur or upper tibia). They are usually considered benign neoplasms, although some can be locally aggressive and some metastasize.

Secondary Tumours

Cancers that commonly metastasise to bone include Breast, Thyroid, Renal, Bronchus and Prostate (not necessarily in this order, but it may help to remember the words "Bone Tumours are Rarely Bony Primaries"). The majority of metastases are lytic lesions, with the exception of prostate, which is usually osteosclerotic (however, breast and thyroid are sometimes osteosclerotic). They metastasise to bone that contains red marrow, otherwise known as the axial skeleton (spine, pelvis, ribs and the proximal end of the long bones).

Secondary tumours may cause local pain or present as a pathological fracture. Pathological fractures are best treated by internal fixation, as they tend not to heal. By the time there are bony secondaries the prognosis is poor and treatment is essentially palliative. Radiotherapy is often used to treat local bone pain.

BONE INFECTION

Infection of bone (osteomyelitis) can be disastrous and extremely difficult to treat, and this is why such meticulous asepsis is undertaken in orthopaedic theatres and why antibiotic prophylaxis is always used when metalwork is involved. Acute osteomyelitis occurs either as a result of haematogenous spread or following trauma/operation. Infection of bones or joints acquired via the blood is common in children but rare in adults, who usually acquire the infection as a result of trauma or operation; the exception to this is in adults who are immunocompromised (including diabetics and those on steroids) or are intravenous drug abusers.

In acute haematogenous osteomyelitis, the usual organisms are *Staphylococcus aureus*, but occasionally streptococci or coliforms are responsible. They enter the blood in many ways, such as via a small skin abrasion or from an infected throat, and settle randomly on the bone.

The symptoms usually include pain and fever, often with a preceding history of either a sore throat or a superficial cut, etc. The limb is painful to move, and there is tenderness and possibly localized inflammation. Diagnosis can be difficult in a young child, who may simply look unwell and have a temperature. X-rays are normal for the first week or so, and later may show a hazy edge to the bone, indicating a periosteal reaction and new bone formation. A bone scan will show up increased activity while the X-rays are still normal.

Bloods should be sent for culture and white cell count, ESR and C-reactive protein (CRP), which should all be raised.

Treatment is by intravenous antibiotics, analgesia and rest of the affected limb. The antibiotics are usually changed to oral after a few days and given for up to six weeks.

Postoperative osteomyelitis where metalwork is *in situ* can be a disaster. Intravenous antibiotics are given and the metalwork may need to be removed and perhaps an external fixator applied if the fracture has not healed.

Chronic osteomyelitis can result if a sequestrum forms. This is an area of pus that is walled off by new bone, often discharging through a sinus. The infection can remain for many years, giving recurrent acute flare-ups. Surgery to remove the sequestrum is indicated if healing is to ensue.

Acute Septic Arthritis

This usually affects large joints such as the hip in children and the knee in adults. The patient will feel unwell, often with a fever and rigors. The joint is painful, inflamed and swollen, and all movements are restricted.

X-rays may be normal initially and an ultrasound may show a joint effusion. Diagnosis can only be made by aspirating the affected joint under aseptic conditions and sending the aspirate to bacteriology for microscopy and culture.

Bloods should include an FBC, ESR, CRP and cultures (do not forget that TB can be a cause).

If the aspirate confirms sepsis, treatment involves joint wash-out under general anaesthetic and IV antibiotics. If there is a prosthesis *in situ*, then the infection may settle only if the metalwork is removed.

Sometimes it is difficult to make a diagnosis, for example when the patient has an acute monoarthritis and the aspirate shows lots of white cells but no organisms. The differential diagnosis includes an acute monoarthritis (rheumatoid), gout, pseudogout, etc. However, clues from the history should help. Does the patient feel generally well or unwell, is he diabetic or on steroids, has he had any previous episodes, etc.? If the blood markers are all normal and the patient looks well, septic arthritis is unlikely and he can be treated with splintage, rest and nonsteroidal, anti-inflammatory drugs. If any doubt as to the diagnosis exists, then he should be admitted for further investigation.

NERVE INJURIES

These are very common in finals and can appear both in medical and in surgical exams. It is worth noting here how you can assess the power of a particular muscle group using the MRC classification, which scores power from 0 to 5; 5 is normal power, 4 is weakness, 3 is ability to use muscle against gravity, 2 is movement with gravity eliminated (for example, able to move in a horizontal direction but not vertically), 1 is just a flicker of the muscle, and 0 means no movement detectable. Despite being quite subjective this is the best clinical method available.

Brachial plexus lesions can be of the upper or lower roots. The closer the lesion is to the spinal cord, the worse the prognosis will be.

Lesions of the upper brachial plexus (Erbs palsy, C5/C6) often occur at birth, and the abductors and external rotators are paralysed, so the arm is held close to the body, internally rotated ("waiter's tip" position), with loss of sensation to the C5/6 dermatomes.

RADIAL NERVE   **ULNAR NERVE**   **MEDIAN NERVE**

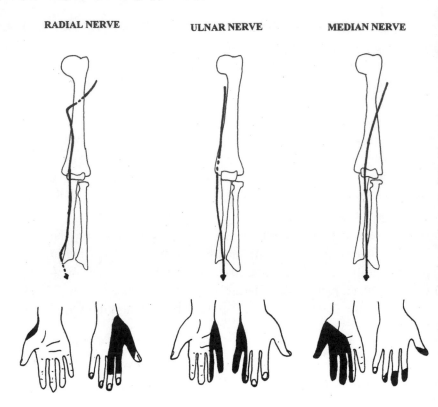

Figure 15.15. Distribution of the peripheral nerves to the arms. The shaded areas on the hands correspond to the sensory distribution of each nerve.

Lesions to the lower brachial plexus (Klumpke paralysis, C8/T1) are rare and result in loss of intrinsic muscles of the hand, leading to a claw hand with loss of sensation in C8/T1 dermatomes.

Injuries to the individual nerves of the arm can occur anywhere along the course of the nerve, and the deficit will depend on the level.

Radial Nerve

Low lesions can occur with fractures around the elbow or forearm, and there is loss of extension of the carpophalangeal joints.

High lesions are more common and usually follow a fracture of the humerus (the nerve is stretched but rarely severed) or after a prolonged tourniquet time. Damage usually occurs where the nerve travels around the shaft of the humerus (radial groove).

The patient has wrist drop, due to paralysis of wrist extensors and loss of sensation along the radial nerve distribution (a common case in finals). The triceps still functions normally.

Very high lesions can be caused by pressure in the axilla (crutches, or Saturday night palsy, where the arm is hung over a chair when the person is drunk and he wakes up with a palsy). This leads to paralysis of triceps as well.

The radial nerve is essentially the nerve which extends the fingers, the wrist and the elbow, and therefore testing the extension of each of these will give a clue as to the level. Sensation is not very accurate in helping to elicit the level, as it is predominantly a motor nerve.

Ulnar Nerve

Damage usually occurs at the elbow or the wrist. The usual picture is a "clawlike hand". The reason for this is that the ulnar nerve supplies half of the flexor digitorum profundus (FDP), the lumbricals to the ring and little fingers and all of the interossei.

A lesion at the wrist causes unopposed action of the extensors and the FDP, especially of the little and ring fingers, causing them to claw (the FDP is supplied just below the elbow and so a cut at the level of the wrist will not paralyse this).

Lesions at the elbow often have less clawing, since the ulnar half of FDP is now paralysed and the fingers are therefore straighter (a true claw hand is seen in Volkman's contracture and proximal lesions of the brachial plexus).

Another test for the ulnar nerve is to ask the patient to grip a piece of paper between the thumb and the proximal phalanx of the index finger of a closed fist. In an ulnar nerve lesion he is unable to use adductor pollicis, and to cheat he flexes the DIPJ using the flexor pollicis (supplied by the median nerve) to grip the paper. If he flexes the DIPJ, then this is a positive Froment's sign.

The sensation in the ulnar distribution of the hand is usually affected. There may be wasting of the interossei on the dorsum of the hand, and there is weakness of finger abduction and adduction.

Therefore, in the short cases, if you see a wrist drop think of the radial nerve, and if you see a claw hand think of the ulnar nerve. Median nerve palsy is usually at the wrist, as in carpal tunnel syndrome.

Carpal Tunnel Syndrome

The median nerve is compressed as it passes under the flexor retinaculum (in the carpal tunnel). It is much more common in females than in males and the associations are pregnancy, rheumatoid arthritis, hypothyroidism, acromegaly and trauma, although most often it is idiopathic in menopausal women. The classic symptoms are pain and paraesthesia in the distribution of the median nerve (see Figure 15.15). A small patch of skin over the thenar eminence is spared, because this is supplied by the superficial branch of the median nerve, which does not go under the flexor retinaculum. The pain is classically worse at night when the patient wakes with pain and tingling in the fingers, which may be relieved by shaking the hands. During the day symptoms may be brought on by activities that compress the nerve further, such as prolonged flexion of the wrist (e.g. typing or knitting). In advanced cases the muscles supplied by the median nerve (often called LOAF muscles) may be weak and wasted. These are the first two Lumbricals and the thenar eminence muscles (Opponens pollicis, Abductor and Flexor pollicis brevis). Ideally diagnosis should be made early from the history, before any physical signs are present. A test that can sometimes reproduce the symptoms is Tinel's test (tapping over the median nerve at the wrist). Always keep in mind a cervical rib or cervical spondylosis involving the C6 & C7 roots, which can cause similar symptoms, although the pain at night is really characteristic of carpal tunnel syndrome. If a case is suspected, diagnosis can be confirmed by electromyographic studies across the wrist showing delayed conduction of the nerve impulses. Treatment can be conservative, by using splints across the wrist or local steroid injections; or surgical, where the tunnel is decompressed by dividing the flexor retinaculum.

Dupuytren's Contracture

This is a common short case or short answer question. Named after the Frenchman who described it in 1931, Guillaine Dupuytren, it is a disorder where there is fibrosis and thickening of the palmar fascia (not the tendons!). It is commoner in men, usually of middle to elderly age. The aetiology is not known, although it can be inherited as an autosomal dominant gene. The associations include alcohol, drugs (such as phenytoin), cirhossis and diabetes.

The condition often begins as a single nodule (which may or may not be painful). Later, bands of thickened tissue form on the palmar fascia which may adhere to the skin and there is progressive contracture of the fingers, usually the ring finger first, followed by the little finger, eventually to the point where the fingers are fully flexed. The condition can be bilateral and the feet can sometimes be affected.

Operation is considered for progressive lesions where the hand can no longer be placed flat on a table. It usually involves a fasciectomy, where the palmar fascia is divided. The condition can, however, recur.

If you see this as a short case, the diagnosis is usually obvious although the differential diagnosis could include a skin contracture (an old laceration, scar or burn is, however, usually visible).

Ganglion

This is a common short case. A ganglion is a cystic swelling, most commonly seen on the dorsum of the wrist. Its exact origin is debated but is probably a cystic mucoid degeneration of the joint capsule or tendon sheath. It usually presents as a painless lump (but it can be painful) that may interfere with wearing a watch or may catch on clothes. A ganglion can disappear spontaneously, although a bash with a Bible was the traditional treatment. It is smooth and fluctuant, and those at the wrist are usually fixed to deeper structures but not to skin. It can be aspirated (thick, gellike material) and injected with hydrocortisone, although it commonly recurs, in which case it can be surgically excised. Again the diagnosis is usually obvious, but the differential, we suppose, could be a lipoma, fibroma or sebaceous cyst.

THE LIMPING CHILD

Paediatric orthopaedics is a postgraduate subject and is not really considered fair game for surgical finals, although you should know a little about the following.

There is a diagnostic calendar of conditions that affect the hip. The following conditions tend to affect the following age groups:

0 (birth):	Congenital dislocation
0–5:	Infections
5–10:	Perthes' disease (Legg–Calve–Perthes')
10–15:	Slipped femoral epiphysis
Adults:	Osteoarthritis, avascular necrosis and rheumatoid

The commonest cause of the painful hip in a child is a transient synovitis secondary to a viral illness, often called the irritable hip.

Congenital Dislocation of the Hip

At birth most hips are stable; however, a small number are dislocated or dislocatable. Most become stable within about two or three weeks. The incidence of congenital dislocation of the hip (CDH) is about 2 per 1000 live births. Females are affected more than males and one-third are bilateral.

The exact aetiology is unknown but there is a familial tendency and there is a high incidence of both joint laxity and a shallow acetabulum in first order relatives of CDH patients. The position of the foetus may play a part as there is a higher incidence in breech presentation.

It is interesting to note that the incidence is much higher in North American Indians, who wrap their babies tight to the mother's body with the hips extended and the legs together, compared to the racially identical Eskimos, who carry their babies on the back with the hips widely abducted and flexed.

The diagnosis should be made at birth, during the routine postnatal examination. Two tests are performed. In *Ortolani's test* the hips and knees are flexed to 90° and the thighs are grasped in each hand, the thumb over the inner thigh and the fingers resting over the greater trochanters. The hips are abducted gently and a resistance to abduction will be noted if the hip is dislocated, otherwise they abduct easily to 90°. When gentle pressure is applied to the greater trochanters by the fingers, a dislocated hip will relocate back into the joint and a click can be felt (positive Ortolani test). *Barlow's test* is a slight modification of this test. It is performed as above except during the abduction phase; gentle but firm pressure is applied in the line of the femur so that a lax hip dislocates posteriorly. The hip pressure can then be reduced by performing the movement in Ortolani's test. Therefore, Ortolani's test detects a dislocated hip and Barlow's test detects a dislocatable hip.

If either test is positive, then the baby should have an ultrasound to show the shape of the cartilaginous socket and the position of the head of the femur. X-rays are not helpful as the femoral head does not start to calcify until about 10 weeks.

Treatment depends on the time of diagnosis, and the sooner the CDH is picked up the easier it is to treat. The aim of treatment is essentially to reduce the hip and hold the head of the femur in this position until the acetabular rim is sufficiently developed.

In the new-born this is achieved initially with double nappies to abduct the hips, and if still unstable after about three weeks an abduction splint can be used which holds the legs abducted, the most popular being the Pavlik harness. The child should be closely monitored with ultrasound and clinical examination for about three months or until the hip is stable.

If a CDH is not picked up at birth but in the next few months, then the same principles apply. However, the dislocation is usually managed by traction and an abduction plaster in a position in which the hip is most stable. After about six months X-rays can be used to assess the acetabulum.

If the CDH is "missed", then diagnosis may not be made until the age of 12–18 months, when the child begins to walk with an abnormal gait. There may be limb shortening, external rotation of the foot, asymmetrical skin creases and a positive Trendelenburg's test. Reduction of the hip in this age group can be achieved by either open or closed methods (although a lip of labrum or loose capsule often impedes reduction and so closed reduction is usually unsuccessful). Open reduction may involve a derotation osteotomy (in order to increase the surface of the head covered by acetabulum, the leg is rotated to a position where the head has maximum covering in the acetabulum; the femur is then sawed just below the trochanters and the shaft allowed to rotate back to a neutral position, and the two ends are then fixed using a plate) and/or an adductor tenotomy (cutting the adductor tendons to decrease the adducting forces on the femur). Once in a good position the hip is held there using a plaster spica.

The prognosis is good if the dislocation is picked up early, although if left untreated it can lead to progressive deformity and disability. With bilateral dislocations the deformity and waddling gait are symmetrical and not so noticeable; in fact such patients often carry on with their lives without much complaint. If you interfere with both sides you run the risk of one side failing and hence converting them to a unilateral asymmetrical deformity, and so most surgeons would not operate on such patients above the age of six.

Perthe's Disease

This is a type of osteochondritis, since it is an avascular necrosis of the femoral head. The patient is usually a male, between 5 and 10 years old, who limps and complains of pain in the hip. Early on all movements are painful, making it difficult to differentiate from infection or a transient synovitis, which is by far the commonest cause of the irritable hip.

Initially X-rays are normal, although a bone scan may show an abnormality. The earliest change to be seen on an X-ray is increased density of the bony part of the epiphysis, which later on flattens and fragments.

Treatment is initially bed rest until the pain subsides, and further operative treatment will depend on the X-rays but essentially involves trying to contain the head in the acetabulum to enable it to retain as good a shape as possible.

Slipped Capital Femoral Epiphysis

Slipped capital femoral epiphysis (SCFE) is an uncommon condition, usually found in children of pubertal age. It tends to affect two contrasting groups, one being the fat and sexually underdeveloped group and the other being the tall and thin group — boys more than girls.

SCFE is thought to be due perhaps to a hormonal imbalance at the time of a growth spurt. The epiphysis slips posteriorly either as an acute event (acute slip) or over a period of time (chronic slip). In an acute slip the patient usually presents with groin pain or pain referred to the thigh or knee. The leg may be slightly short, externally rotated, and initially all movements are painful. Treatment depends on the acuteness of presentation and the degree of displacement but usually involves surgery to reduce the epiphysis and hold it in place with a pin. In a chronic slip, reduction should not be attempted (as avascular necrosis may result) and the epiphysis is usually pinned where it is to prevent further slippage.

Irritable Hip

This is a diagnosis of exclusion commonly made in children between the ages of 1 and 10, and presents with a limp and pain in the hip. The cause is unknown but may be a viral synovitis as the patient often has a preceding upper respiratory tract infection. It is important to rule out septic arthritis, and so screening blood tests, including a full blood count, CRP and ESR, must be sent off. Infection in a joint leads to destruction of the articular crtilage and permanent damage within a short space of time, and therefore a child in whom you suspect infection needs urgent aspiration of the joint to obtain microbiological samples for microscopy and culture.

The irritable hip usually settles with rest and analgesia over two or three days.

16

THE EXAM

Examinations are formidable even to the best prepared, for the greatest
fool may ask more than the wisest man can answer.

— C. C. Colton

Most medical schools set a mixture of written, viva voce and clinical
examinations. Written papers may be essay questions, short answers or
multiple choice questions. Clinical exams consist of either short cases
or long cases, or both. In some medical schools, medical and surgical
cases are examined together. In most, surgical cases are examined in a
separate section of the exam. It is important that you understand how
the exam runs in your own medical school, as it will influence the way
you should prepare for it. You need also to try and find out who the
examiners are and to make particularly sure that you know what their
special interests are. You should speak to people who have done the
exam in previous years and look through as many past papers as possible.

Each year at medical school the majority of students pass their finals.
All that the examiners are really doing is to vet out anyone who clearly
is unsafe to be a houseman. It is a bit like a game with hard and fast
rules. If you abide by the rules of the game you will pass, and if you
break them you may fail. The following list includes some of the rules
concerning how not to fail finals:

- Dress smartly and look respectable.
- Be polite to the patient, and try to build up rapport, because if he
  does not like you he may land you in difficulty.

- Never hurt the patient.
- Never make up anything, and never say anything dangerous. If you do not know something say that you will ask a senior for advice or for a drug say that you would look it up in the *British National Formulary* (*BNF*).
- The examiners are always right — do not answer back and do not argue.

If the examiners think that you are unsafe then they will fail you. Know your emergencies, because if your viva is not going well the examiners will usually change the subject to one that you should know something about in order to be a safe house officer. For example, you should know the emergency management of a shocked patient. If you said you would do a CT scan before placing two large bore venflons in both antecubital fossae and starting fluids, then you would deserve to fail.

WRITTEN PAPERS

It is important to deal with this part of the exam with care and a prepared approach. You should also aim to practise written answers before the exam. Remember that many examiners attach great importance to legibility, accuracy and clearness of expression. In most universities answers have to be written into specific mark books and there are often requirements to write candidate numbers on each page, start each answer on a new sheet, etc. Try to follow these instructions in full. It may be advisable to use alternate lines in an answer book if this improves legibility, and it may also be a good idea to underline section headings, perhaps with a different colour. Use an appropriate pen for written answers and avoid unusual colours of ink. Resist the temptation to write so quickly that your writing becomes illegible.

Essay Questions

Try to get some practice in essay writing before the exam. Writing an essay to a time limit is a definite skill which can be enormously improved with practice. It is obvious that one should read the questions carefully before starting to answer the paper, but it is amazing how many students apparently fail to do this. The examiners will usually have decided on an approximate allocation of marks for each point made and discussed. There may be some spare marks to award arbitrarily for excellence but they will be relatively few. What this means is that you will get most of the marks for simply mentioning or sketching out points and relatively few for elaboration. If you spend time answering things which have not been asked for, no matter how good your answer is, there will be no marks. An example would be "How might a peptic ulcer present?" and the candidate spends time discussing how it might be treated. Many medical schools (and postgraduate exams like FRCS or MRCS) use "close marking" schemes. The essence of these is that questions are all given marks close the pass mark, i.e. 40 for a bad fail, 65 for a very good answer. This means that it is very difficult to make up for answers left completely unattempted.

The only way to avoid simple types of error is to have a set plan of approach, since it is so easy to make an error in the heat of battle. We would suggest the following:

- Read the instructions at the top of the paper carefully (i.e. how many questions should be answered, time allowed, etc. Do not presume that they will be the same as for past papers you may have looked at during your revision). If you are not sure ask the invigilator, who is there for that purpose.
- Calculate exactly how much time should be spent on each question after allowing five minutes for reading the paper and five minutes for each essay plan.
- Slowly read each question in turn, until you are sure you understand what it is asking.
- Spend five minutes on each question thinking and then writing a rough plan. Use the surgical sieve to help you not forget anything. Do all the plans first.
- Only then start writing the essays themselves. Start with the one you feel you can answer best.

- Spend only the amount of time allowed on any one question.
- On no account fail to answer all questions. If the worst happens and you run out of time, hand in your essay plan.

Multiple Choice Questions

The basic way most multiple choice exams are marked is that you get one mark for a correct answer, nothing for an answer not attempted and one mark is taken away for an incorrect answer. This means that guesswork is unlikely to improve your marks and may in fact reduce them, since questions may be deliberately misleading.

We suggest you approach the multiple choice in the following way:

- Calculate the time available and aim to go through the paper in 60% of that time.
- Go through answering only the questions you are fairly certain you know the answers to.
- Make sure you spend a moment on each question considering the exact wording and sense of the question — this can make a big difference in the multiple choice. For example, "perforated peptic ulcer is always treated by operation" is not the same as "perforated peptic ulcer is usually treated by operation".
- Go back over the questions you have not answered and see if there are any that you can now answer with a fair degree of certainty.
- Questions using the words *always* and *never* are invariably false; likewise questions using the word *may* are usually true (for example, "vomiting is *always* present in bowel obstruction" — false).
- Leave questions unanswered when your answer would be complete guesswork.
- Some MCQ's are not negatively marked and for these you should answer all the questions, even if you have to guess.

Short Answer Questions

Even more than with essay questions the examiners will be awarding marks on the basis of individual points mentioned. Once again there will be few marks which can be flexibly awarded and no marks for points in the answer which do not address the question as actually asked. It is usually not necessary (or possible time-wise) to do a plan, but in many ways the answers should have the obvious structure of a plan anyway. As with essay questions you should first of all spend five minutes reading the instructions and all the questions twice. Then decide which questions you are going to answer and calculate the time to be spent on each question. Do not spend more time on any one question and make sure you finish all the questions.

CLINICAL EXAMINATION

This is often the most worrying part of the exam for students. It is often difficult to think clearly in such a high tension situation and it is important that you have prepared your basic history-taking and examining techniques in advance so that you can perform these on "auto-pilot" and concentrate specifically on your answers to the examiners. You should be smartly dressed and arrive early.

Viva Voce Examination

This usually takes the form of the candidate sitting at a desk opposite two examiners. Topics can cover any area of surgery, and sometimes X-rays, specimens or surgical instruments may be shown. In some medical schools the viva is the last part of the exam and then commonly the examiners will know something of the candidates' performance to that point. In other medical schools the viva is only held for deciding who should get a distinction or for those with borderline marks who are in some danger of failing.

The examiners develop an overall impression of you; therefore, it is important not to ponder over the first question asked. If you do not understand a question, after a short period of reflection tell the examiners that you do not understand and ask them to rephrase the question. If you do this they will usually give some extra information or a hint to help you in the correct direction. This is much better than simply asking them to repeat the question when you will probably get no extra information and will still be unable to answer. Remember, if the questions appear to be getting harder this usually means you are doing well, as the examiners need to assess how good you are, so that they can give you a grade. Most people leave the room only remembering the last question asked — which is, as explained, usually the most difficult. This is why you should never ask the candidate leaving the viva before you what he was asked.

Short Cases

The examiners usually work in pairs, with one questioning and the other marking. Do not be put off by this. There is no truth in the commonly held belief that you have to get through a particular number of short cases to be able to pass. Remember to briefly introduce yourself to the patient, ask him if he minds you examining him and preserve his dignity when examining him but do not compromise on exposure. Most marks will be awarded for using the correct technique of examination and not necessarily for reaching a diagnosis. Not all short cases will take the same length of time to deal with. If the case is very straightforward (for example a case of Dupuytren's) simply state the features and diagnosis so that the examiners can either move on or ask you extra questions about treatment, etc. Above all, be guided by the examiners as to what you should examine and how quickly.

Common short cases include neck lumps (especially thyroid), groin lumps (especially hernias and testicular lumps), hands (Dupytren's, ganglions and nerve lesions), skin cancer and lumps (e.g. lipomata and neufibromata), abdominal examinations (enlarged liver or stomas), orthopaedic cases (especially knees and feet) and varicose veins.

Long Cases

Most medical schools expect the candidate to be examined on a surgical long case. The principle of the long case is that the candidate is left alone with the patient to take a history and carry out an examination. Leave five minutes at the end to quickly gather your thoughts on how you are going to present the case to the examiners. The time allowed with the patient varies from twenty minutes to one hour. In medical schools where one hour is allowed, this is usually enough time for a full standard history and examination, and time itself should pose no problem. When the time is shorter, the candidate may have to limit the history and examination to the most important points. This will be understood by the examiners, and if asked about something you have not had time to do, you must state this clearly. It is a fatal error to waffle or, even worse, make something up. Remember also that the examiners may take you back to the case and go over the points in question with you. If you are found to have made something up, then usually you will automatically fail. If possible present the case without looking at your notes all the time (sample presentations are given at the back of the book). Eye contact with the examiners will help to make a good impression.

Common long cases include abdominal operations (e.g. postop bowel resection for cancer or inflammatory bowel disease), vascular cases (carotid disease, aortic aneurysm or peripheral vascular disease), orthopaedic cases (joint replacements for osteoarthritis) and breast lumps (usually elderly patients).

Objective Structured Clinical Exams (OSCE's)

Many medical schools are now introducing OSCE's as part of their examinations. The principle of these is to provide uniformity in the exam for all students and not have the unpredictabilty that is inherent in the standard clinical exams. Since all candidates will face the same clinical problems, it is possible to unify marking across examiners in a way that would not otherwise be possible. Often actors are used instead of real patients. The usual approach for an OSCE exam is to have a number of "stations" at which the candidate has to carry out tasks. For example, one station might be to carry out an abdominal exam, another to consent a patient for a colostomy, etc. Examiners are present to mark the candidate, which can sometimes be off-putting; however, they would not normally speak or question the candidate directly. Some stations may also consist of X-rays with a list of questions, pictures of clinical signs, etc., in which the candidate completes an answer sheet which is marked afterwards.

There is nothing inherent in an OSCE examination which should trouble the well-prepared candidate. One problem can be completing the task within the time allowed at each station, and you should therefore find out the format of the exam well in advance and practise doing things to time.

APPENDIX

SAMPLE LONG CASE CLERKINGS

When you present your long case to your examiner, have a provisional diagnosis or differential in your mind. It is sometimes possible to predict what questions the examiner is going to ask you, and it will help if you have thought of the answers before the question is asked. Here are some sample presentations from real finals cases. Note that they are concise and contain only the relevant facts. Leave five minutes at the end of your clerking to get your ideas together and to write a quick summary.

CASE 1

Mr J. S. is a 67-year-old retired builder. He has attended today for the purpose of the exams. He presents with a year's history of progressive pain in his left hip. Over the last three months, however, the pain has worsened, and it now interferes with his sleep. He occasionally needs a stick and has particular difficulty in climbing stairs. Whereas in the past he could walk long distances, he can now only walk 200 yards before he is limited by pain in the groin and he also has difficulty in putting on his shoes and socks. His GP prescribed Ibuprofen, which despite some initial help is now of no use.

There has been no history of trauma and he denies any problems with his other joints. He is married and lives in a two-storey house with his wife.

In his past medical history he had an appendicectomy at age 12 but otherwise has been fit and well, with no cardiorespiratory disease. He has no relevant family history and his only medication is Ibuprofen. He denies any allergies and does not smoke or drink.

On systems review the only positive findings were those of prostatism, where he reports nocturia twice nightly, a poor stream, and terminal dribbling of his urine.

On examination he is slightly overweight (weighing 110 kg, with a height of five foot six. [If you could work out the body mass index, you certainly would impress the examiners. NB: BMI = weight^2 (kg)/height (cm) and is normally under 25.] But he looks generally well, with no signs of anaemia, jaundice or lymphadenopathy.

Cardiorespiratory examination was unremarkable (have it written, in case they ask you about any particular point), and abdominal examination revealed an appendicectomy scar but the patient was otherwise normal. I did not perform a rectal examination but would normally do so, to feel the size and consistency of his prostate. On examination of his hips he has an antalgic gait with a positive Trendelenburg's test. There was no leg length discrepancy. He has a fixed flexion deformity of 10° on the left side and a decreased range of movement of the left hip (flexion 10–85, abduction 35, adduction 10, internal rotation 10 and external rotation 15°). The movements were most painful in full flexion and internal rotation. Examination of the right hip, the back and both knees was normal.

There was no neurovascular deficit and no signs of peripheral vascular or venous disease.

In summary, this 67-year-old retired builder has a year's history of progressively worsening pain in his left hip which is now affecting his lifestyle and ability to sleep at night. My provisional diagnosis is that of osteoarthritis.

The examiners will then ask what investigations you would like to perform (plain X-rays) and will make you comment on them. They are likely to ask you about anything you have said.

If your diagnosis is correct, then the questions they may ask you are as follows:

(1) What is the treatment? (Conservative vs surgical — lose weight, physio, etc., although the patient will probably need a hip replacement.)

(2) You say in your history that he has prostatism — is that relevant? (Yes, he may go into postoperative retention.)

(3) The examiners may talk to the patient and ask you about your positive findings. [Trendelenburg's test, leg length, fixed flexion (Thomas's test).]

CASE 2

Mrs J. P. is a 51-year-old housewife who is currently an in-patient at this hospital, awaiting surgery. She presents with a lump in her left breast. She first noticed the lump two weeks ago whilst showering and it has not changed since then. She has no symptoms from the lump and she had never noticed any breast lumps before. Her main concern is that this is a cancer.

Her menarche was at age 12 and her periods were always regular up until her menopause two years ago. She has been on hormone replacement therapy since. She has had no children through her own and her husband's wishes, and she has no family history of breast cancer.

She went to her GP, who sent her to the breast clinic last week, where she underwent a needle test and a mammography. She says the results were suggestive of cancer and she has been admitted for surgery.

She has no relevant past medical history and is on no medication, but is allergic to penicillin, which gives her a rash. She lives with her husband, smokes 10 cigarettes a day and drinks only occasionally.

Systems review was negative for any problems in the cardiovascular, respiratory, abdominal and neurological systems.

On examination she looks well and is not pale or jaundiced.

Examination of her breasts reveals that both nipples are inverted, although she says this has been present for as long as she can remember. She has a 3 cm hard lump in the upper outer quadrant of her left breast. The lump has an irregular outline but is mobile and not tethered to the chest wall or the skin. She has no lymphadeno-pathy and no evidence of metastatic spread on examination of her abdomen, chest and spine. Cardiorespiratory examination was unremarkable.

In summary, this 51-year-old postmenopausal lady has a suspicious 3 cm lump in her left breast. She has undergone triple assessment in the clinic and has been admitted for surgery tomorrow.

The examiners will ask questions like:

(1) What is your differential diagnosis? [Benign or malignant, etc. Cancer, fat necrosis, fibroadenoma (rare in this age group).]
(2) If you saw this lady in the clinic what investigations would you perform? (Triple assessment.)
(3) Are there any further investigations that can be performed? (Trucut and staging procedures.)
(4) What treatments are available?

INDEX

A

B

I

S